50 Ways to Boost Your Metabolism

Fredrik Paulún

Translated by **Ellen Hedström**

Skyhorse Publishing

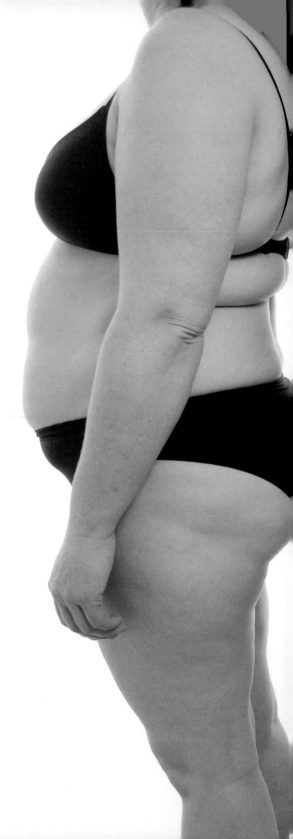

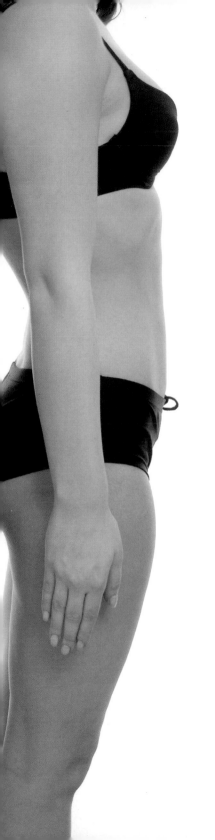

50 Ways to Boost Your Metabolism

Fredrik

Paulún

Translated by   **Ellen Hedström**

Contents

Introduction

Eat Your Way to Better Fat Burning

Drink Efficiently and Burn Fat

Spices That Boost Your Metabolism

Nutrients, Hormones, and Other Bits and Pieces

Feel Great and Increase Your Metabolism

Introduction

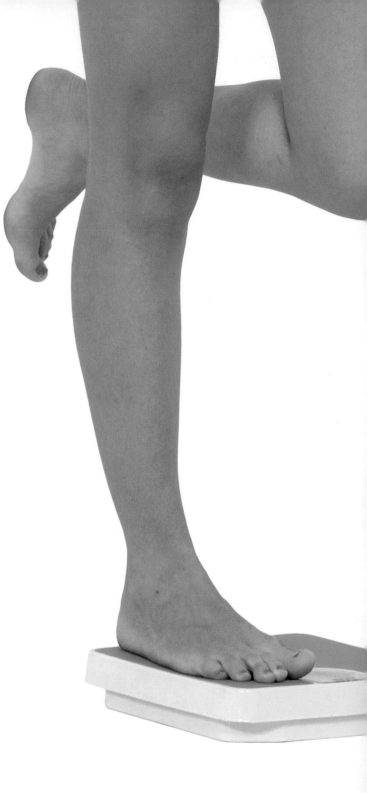

Let's Start at the Beginning

You're holding a book filled with easy-to-follow hints to boost your metabolism and improve your ability to burn fat. My shortcuts are perfect for anyone who wants to reduce body fat or learn how to enhance the effect of his or her current diet. These tips boost all diets, but you don't need to be on a diet to experience the benefits of this book!

All of the advice in the following pages is based on the latest scientific research. The numbers that appear in parentheses throughout the text refer to scientific studies that demonstrate the points I make.

These shortcuts work for several reasons. They might increase your metabolism, slow down the uptake of calories (or even reduce them), or increase the rate at which you burn fat. But the results are always the same: They reduce the body's tendency to store fat. So, choose the tips that work for your body and your lifestyle. The more you embrace them, the better the effects.

In essence, losing weight is about burning more calories than you consume. But that's not all—you must have a good metabolism because it's fat that you want to lose, not muscle. The ways to get a quick metabolism can vary in practice, but the easiest and healthiest is to increase the rate at which you expend energy, rather than dramatically reducing your food intake. A slight decrease in your energy intake is fine, but if you dip too low, your body will respond by reducing the basal metabolic rate, meaning you will lose too much muscle.

What Determines Metabolism?

What is it that determines how much energy you use? Some would guess that it has to do with age, sex, weight, height, and so on. But in truth, these aren't determining factors. Heavier people do tend to use up more energy, but there are other factors that rule first and foremost.

Basal Energy Expenditure

Basal energy expenditure is the basic energy usage required to stay alive, even when at complete rest. Even if you are lying completely still, staring only at the ceiling, your heart, lungs, and cells still need energy. The cells, for example, pump salt back and forth; this action goes completely unnoticed by you, but you would die if it ceased, and this action takes energy.

The amount of the basal energy expenditure varies somewhat, but it is generally between 1100-1300 kcal a day. It can sink with starvation and diet, but basal energy expenditure rarely goes below 800 kcal per day.

> kcal = kilocalories, but these are usually known as "calories," which is the term used in this book.

Physical Activity

As you might have guessed, this is about the work that your muscles do. It can be anything from playing computer games to running, and even the smallest effort—such as getting out of bed—counts. So it comes as no surprise that it is this part of energy expenditure that varies the most between individuals. It can range from zero or a few hundred kcal for a physically disabled person to up to 5000 kcal for a super endurance athlete. So, for anyone who wants to lose weight, this is a good place to start. There is a lot here that you yourself can influence, and each little effort counts; this is why day-to-day exercise is so important. If you take the stairs instead of the elevator, park the car a ten-minute walk from your workplace, or even stand rather than sit on the bus, you will easily burn an extra hundred calories a day. Over a year, that adds up to 36,500 kcal—about the same amount of energy as is contained in 11 lb (5 kg) of body fat.

Heat Production

Producing heat is a necessity for all warm-blooded creatures because we need to keep our body temperature up. The production of heat—thermogenesis—is so vital that it is constantly working, even coping with regulating body temperature during cold weather. So, despite many suggestions to the contrary, cold weather doesn't normally increase metabolism.

It's only when it's so cold that you start to shiver that the production of heat actually increases. Shivering is a result of the muscles contracting and relaxing, and this involuntary movement heats the body. After a longer period of cold (which is unhealthy because it increases the risk of disease-causing viruses and bacteria), the body can maintain increased production of heat more constantly because your *brown fat* increases its energy consumption. Brown fat can be found in the upper parts of the breast and neck area, and its main task is to produce heat. It gets its name from the color created by the large amounts of mitochondria (known as the power station of the cells) as they convert fat to heat.

Warm weather, on the other hand, can raise the basal energy expenditure by up to 10 percent because the heart has to work harder, and superficial blood vessels need to dilate in order for heat to leave the body.

One type of thermogenesis known as *mealtime induced thermogenesis* is the increase of body temperature that occurs after a meal. This occurs in part due to the actual digestion of food and partly because of metabolism. Storage is a third reason because as energy is required to store carbohydrates in the form of glucose. Tests have shown that on average 0-3 percent of the energy contained in fat evaporates after a meal. Compare this to 5-10 percent for carbohydrates, or as much as 20-30 percent for proteins, so there really is a difference among the nutrients.

People with a lowered sensitivity to insulin tend to have a lower temperature increase, which can affect weight. For example, if the metabolism is reduced by 150 kcal per day, this is equal to the energy contained in around 16 lb (7.5 kg) of body fat in a year.

Growth

Growth is the third aspect of energy expenditure—for those who are growing, that is. This includes children, pregnant women, athletes who are building muscle, and those who are gaining weight. This is the energy that remains after you have covered your basal need, your physical activity, and your heat production, and it goes to weight gain. If you increase your physical activity (e.g., by taking daily walks), or your heat production (by a generous consumption of strong spices), less will go to growth, and you will be better able to maintain your weight.

Metabolism vs. Fat Burning

Many people use the terms *metabolism* and *fat burning* loosely and get them confused. These words do not actually denote the same thing, even if they are related. The term "to burn" is used by many when describing energy expenditure, but this is not entirely correct.

Fat burning is the process by which your cells burn fat, and it is burning fat that converts a handful of nuts to a few running strides in your cells' power station: the mitochondria. An increased ability to burn fat, therefore, means that you consume several grams more fat per hour than before, but it doesn't automatically mean that your metabolism has increased. If, for example, you should experience starvation, your consumption of energy would decrease to conserve energy. In this scenario, because there is essentially no other source of energy but fat and some protein for your body to use, the rate of fat burning would increase, but your metabolism would decrease. Almost 90 percent of your metabolism is covered by fat burning.

For those who want to keep their body fat low and stay in shape, it would be optimal to increase energy expenditure with the help of exercise and a better diet, and to increase the amount of fat that is burned. This will result in both a reduction in body fat as well as more energy for workouts. This is what the tips in this book refer to.

Energy expenditure is the sum of the four factors that we have just covered: basal energy expenditure, physical activity, heat production, and growth. Metabolism describes the conversion of nutrients in your body.

Energy Intake

Everything you eat and drink that contains calories gives you a certain amount of energy and contributes to your energy intake. The body is generally very good at making sure you take in as much energy as you need (the same amount that you expend). However, sometimes mistakes are made.

Appetite is a very complex phenomenon, which is regulated by how full the stomach feels, body temperature, and the accessibility of nutrients in the blood. Most of what regulates appetite occurs in the brain: in areas such as the hypothalamus, the diencephalon, and the cerebral cortex. Other organs involved in regulating appetite are the liver, fat tissue, and the gut. These systems were developed during prehistoric times when there was a completely different diet from today's, so modern, refined foods with a high energy content—quick pasta, ready meals, chips, etc.—make it easy to overeat. The unfortunate fact is that a small surplus of energy will, over time, cause steady and substantial weight gain. You might as well raise your eyebrows when I tell you that 90 percent of those who gain weight could completely avoid this by consuming 50 kcal fewer per day (162). And 50 kcal is about the energy content of an apple!

Naturally, this surplus of energy can be compensated for by taking a walk of about half a mile (1 km) or so, or even eating a couple fewer mouthfuls at each meal. I understand that this is easier said than done, and so it's helpful to find small ways to instantly reduce your energy intake or increase your metabolism. This book was written to help you do exactly this, and I will present you with all the tricks that current research has revealed.

Energy Absorption

More and more, research is showing that we don't actually absorb everything we eat. From a normal portion, up to 10-20 percent of available energy can pass straight through the gut if the food is rich in fiber, contains wholegrain, and has some bite to it. In contrast, a dish of refined fast food that is poor in fiber has an almost 100 percent absorption rate. Obviously, absorbing 100 percent of a meal made up of junk food will have a long-term effect on weight gain. It's important to think about how easily the foods you eat can be digested and to weigh your options carefully because foods that are easier to digest are absorbed more easily. Cooked vegetables, for example, are often better to eat than their raw counterparts because the absorption rate from cooked vegetables is significantly higher. The fiber content is the same, but because the structure of cooked vegetables is more porous, they become easier to digest. Vegetables are poor in energy content, but they are rich in vitamins, minerals, and antioxidants. Therefore, absorbing their nutrients properly is highly beneficial (this is in contrast to low-nutrient dishes like pancakes).

Chewing food properly also increases the amount of energy you can absorb. Chewing carelessly and eating quickly is not helpful because a frantic eating style produces a rise in blood sugars, resulting in fat-building insulin. It also takes a while before you start to feel full from a meal; this means that eating too quickly can easily lead to overeating long before the feeling of being full is able to kick in.

Now it's finally time to get going with the shortcuts. Of course, you can read them in any order you wish, but I would recommend that you at least read through the first shortcut on carbohydrates. It contains a lot of useful information that will further your understanding of many of the other shortcuts.

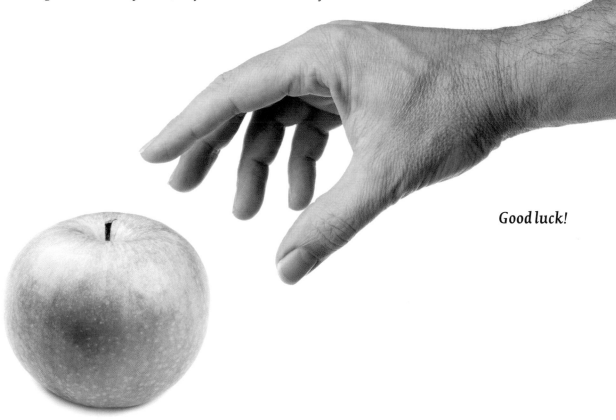

Good luck!

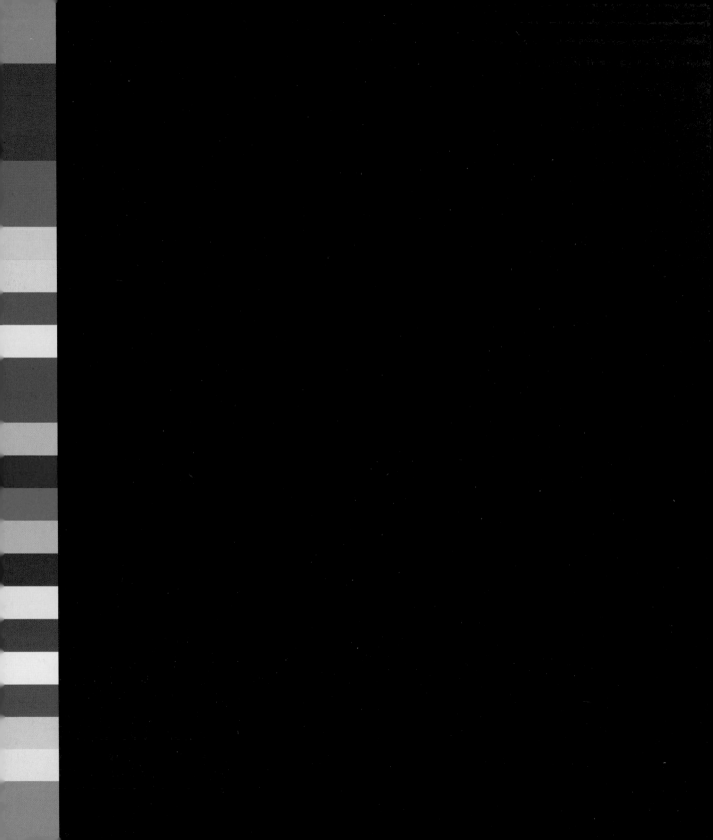

Eat Your Way to Better Fat Burning

Carbohydrates

–Increase or Decrease Your Metabolism

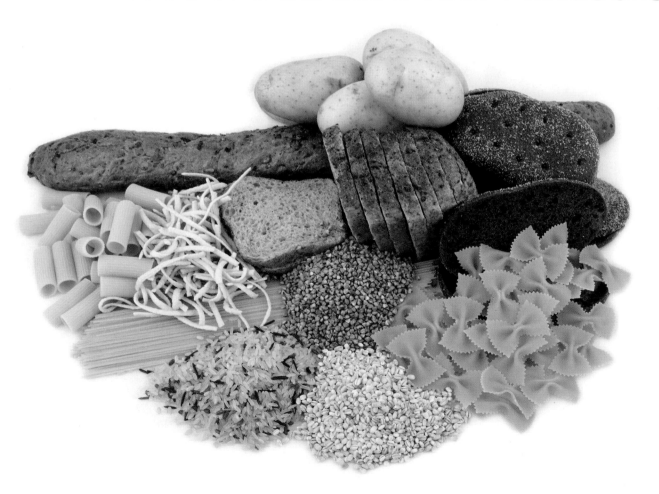

■ Over the past ten years, the benefits of carbohydrates have been increasingly debated. There can't be many who have never heard of GI or LCHF, and the "carb monster" has gotten its claws into many people. It's true that carbohydrates affect weight and well-being, but the effect is simply negative. So, before I offer any advice, I'd like to give you a little background.

Carbohydrates are a fantastic nutrient. They are the brain's favorite fuel, and it alone consumes around 4 to 4 ½ oz (120-130 g) of carbohydrates each day. This is the equivalent of six bananas that your brain thinks away every day! Your muscles and liver also use carbohydrates, and the more you move, the more carbohydrates are used. This is why we need to consume a certain amount of food at each mealtime in order to feel satisfied.

In the body, carbohydrates are converted into blood sugar to be absorbed by the brain, muscles, and liver, but blood sugar (also known as glucose) has another side to it. If your blood contains too much sugar, there is the risk that the blood sugar might get "stuck" to the proteins in your body, which would not be good because the proteins will get damaged and lose function. Simply put, blood sugar binds to proteins that are found in the brain, eyes, blood, veins, muscles, muscle attachments, and so on; this process is known as *glycation*. If glycation occurs slowly—for example, if a person has slightly raised blood sugar levels over several decades—it will speed up the aging process. Dementia, high blood pressure, heart disease, diabetes, and vision problems are all normal signs of aging that can be advanced due, in part, to high blood sugar.

If blood sugar rises too quickly in large amounts, as it might do in type 1 diabetes that has been left untreated, several organs will begin to shut down; this, of course, can be life threatening. This is why the body maintains total control of blood sugar levels and will not let your blood sugar rise too high or dip too low. Blood sugar is both good and essential, but it is vital that it be kept in balance.

Insulin: Your Key to Health and Burning Fat

The tool that the body uses to combat excessively high levels of blood sugar is called *insulin*. Insulin is a hormone that lowers blood sugar and unlocks the liver and muscles to allow blood sugar to be stored inside them. In this manner, you avoid glycation and gain energy in your muscles, strengthening them and building your endurance. The more carbohydrates you eat, the faster they raise your blood sugar, and the more insulin is released. When you binge on a lot of candy, your blood sugar skyrockets, and a huge amount of insulin is released to counter it. The natural consequence of this reaction is that the fast-rising blood sugar will sink again just as rapidly, and as the cells quickly absorb the blood sugar, you'll start to feel hungry again.

In addition, insulin opens the fat cells; the more insulin you have in your blood, the more fat is stored. This is how people can get fat from consuming too many fast-acting carbohydrates.

A moderate insulin level is not only good for weight regulation, but it can even protect against heart disease, type 2 diabetes, premature aging, and many forms of cancer.

When carbohydrates reach the blood and turn into blood sugar, they release insulin and unlock your cells, so that your cells can absorb this blood sugar to use as fuel. It is vital that the correct amount of insulin be released and that it properly unlocks the cells because this will result in balanced blood sugar that never rises to dangerous levels.

The link between insulin (which can be described as a key) and its receptors (the keyholes) on the surface of the cell has to work perfectly. Many people suffer from so-called insulin sensitivity; this can be as a result of inactivity, stress, illness, smoking, lack of sleep, being overweight, eating too many fast-acting carbohydrates, or consuming the wrong fats. Insulin sensitivity means that the "keys" don't work properly, forcing the body to release more insulin than is needed. Consequently, there is too much sugar and insulin in the blood, resulting in the glycation of the blood sugar as well as weight gain (caused by the insulin stimulating the storage of fat).

There is one more hormone that is significant when burning fat and is influenced by the rise in blood sugars after a meal. It is called *adiponectin*, and it can increase fat burning. Foods with slow-acting carbohydrates and those with the right amount of carbohydrates can increase adiponectin (49, 50).

> **Reduced/low sensitivity to insulin:** When the insulin ("the key") doesn't work on the cell's receptors ("the lock") and the body has to release more insulin to compensate. This results in high levels of both insulin and blood sugar.

Slow-Acting Carbohydrates are People Food

Mankind has always eaten slow-acting carbohydrates. This is what our bodies are designed for, and we should continue to do so. The availability of slow-acting carbs today is huge—in both good and bad foods—and it is easy to eat right with a bit of nutritional know-how.

When it comes to carbs, both the quantity and the speed matter. Examples of good sources of carbs are unsweetened bread with wholegrain (preferably sourdough), slow-cooked whole wheat pasta, slow-cooked brown rice, whole grain flakes (such as oat porridge), unsweetened muesli, fruit and vegetables of all varieties (even bananas!), berries, mushrooms, legumes (beans, peas, lentils), nuts, seeds, and root vegetables (even boiled potatoes).

When it comes to carbs, you should eat meat, fish, poultry, eggs, shellfish, oil, avocados, olives, and other foods low in carbs that also give fat and/or protein because they delay the emptying of the stomach and will lead to a slower digestion of the carbs and fats. This means that blood sugar increases more slowly, resulting in a stable blood-sugar curve and a lower production of insulin. You should always mix your meals with all three nutrients, but don't forget: Fruits and vegetables also contain carbs, so you don't need to eat a pile of pasta or potatoes! The iso diet is a good method for portioning your meals so as to reach optimal weight loss and fat burn. You can read more about the iso diet on page 52.

The Glycemic Index: A Useful Tool

As you already know, there is a smart tool that can be used when finding slow-release carbs. It's called the *glycemic index*. If you want to read more about this there are a plethora of books devoted to this subject. Put simply, food with a low GI contains slow-release carbs, and vice versa.

What happens when you eat the right carbs and get the right amount of carbs with a low GI? Several studies show that food with a low GI lead to increased weight loss more than other foods. There are even studies that show that following this method is more effective than more conventional low-calorie diets, even when test subjects could eat as much low GI food as they wanted (52).

> **Glycemic Index:** GI is a measurement of how fast the blood sugar rises after you have eaten about 2 oz (50 g) of carbohydrates (not 2 oz of food). A low GI means slow-release carbs and vice versa.

Avoid Carbs that Inhibit Fat Burning

Sources of carbs that inhibit fat burning are simply those foods that have a high GI value and that contain a larger number of carbs (quantity plays a big part). A small piece of candy will hardly affect your fat burn, but a large bag of it will decrease the burning of fat for hours. Foods that have a high GI and large amounts of carbs include soda, squash, cakes, ice cream, cookies, candy, jams, white bread, quick pasta, quick rice, sushi rice (even if sushi itself is okay), cornflakes, French fries, cheese doodles, and many types of crispy bread (a good, crispy bread will have seeds and/or whole grains in/ on them).

To Remove Carbohydrates Is to Remove Success

To both lower the GI in the food you eat (by consuming slow carbohydrates) and eating slightly fewer carbs is an excellent strategy for stimulating fat burning. To completely remove carbs, such as with an extreme diet like LCHF (low carb high fat), is often less successful for most people because the brain's need for glucose is not met, and the body is left to produce an alternative fuel called *ketone*. Ketone keeps the brain going, but it makes a less efficient fuel than glucose. It's a bit like driving a car with a wood engine: it works, but not very well. In addition, sensitivity to insulin decreases as the body is trying to conserve the glucose for the brain. This means that many of those who follow an LCHF diet have high levels of insulin, even though they have hardly any blood sugar. It's a strange paradox, and over time, it becomes unhealthy. In addition, the body's levels of cortisol and norepinephrine increase when you abstain from consuming carbs. These two hormones assist the body in emptying the store of carbohydrates that are normally contained in the liver, but at the same time, they have a degenerative effect on muscles and your immune system. In addition, cortisol can actually stimulate fat storage, and norepinephrine is a hormone that makes you itchy and irritated—hardly desirable when it comes to quality of life!

Low and Slow Without Carbs

Research shows that if you cut out carbs from your diet, you lower your production of serotonin. One study compared those who removed as many carbs from their diet as possible with those who still consumed carbs here and there. Both groups lost the same amount of weight; however, those who did not eat carbs reported feeling much sadder after the duration of the year-long diet. This was probably due to lower levels of serotonin in the brain (46). Serotonin is our "happy hormone," and it makes us calm and happy, and allows for a good night's sleep. Low serotonin levels can make people aggressive and impulsive.

Also, to remove carbs and replace them with large quantities of fat seems to be bad for heart health because LDL (the bad cholesterol) increases and is a risk factor for heart disease (45). By removing carbs, you decrease your energy and remove the will to work out. Research shows that the more ketones you have in your blood the more strenuous physical activity becomes (46, 47). But we want to exercise to feel good and to increase our metabolism. Of course, people all have slightly different predispositions, but if you eat around

20-30 percent of calories from carbohydrates—for example, from fruit, berries, salads, and root vegetables—you shouldn't have any problems with exercise.

Fructose: A Trickster

GI is clearly a useful tool for losing weight, but you shouldn't get fixated on your blood sugar levels. A tricky type of sugar is *fructose*, which can be found in white sugar, as well in many other products in its pure form. If the content label says fructose and/or corn syrup, that product contains pure fructose. If you eat too much fructose, it can have an unexpected effect: fat storage will increase, even if the GI value is low. The GI is low because fructose itself can become blood sugar, but it has to be converted in the liver, and in this way, it increases blood sugar levels very slowly. However, the liver only stores about 2-2 ½ oz (50-75 g) of glycogen and it will quickly get filled up if too much fructose is ingested. This, in turn, means that the liver will become reluctant to absorb glucose from the blood. The liver overflows, the excess is converted to fat, and the increased amount of glucose in the blood (that which could not be absorbed by the liver) affects the body's sensitivity to insulin. As you may remember, this is a step toward type 2 diabetes. Large consumption of pure fructose, therefore, can increase the storage of fat and increase the risk for serious metabolic illnesses (51). Even glycogen (stored glucose in the liver), lactic acid, and fat are created by fructose, and the more you eat, the more increased the production of fat becomes.

Eating fruit in normal amounts is absolutely fine because these carbs are not so dense. An apple has a teaspoon (5 g) of fructose, which your liver easily has space for and will not cause any negative effect. The antioxidants, fibers, vitamins, minerals, and slow-release carbs have excellent effects on your health and metabolism. Even honey and dried fruit consumed in reasonable quantities are good for your health; it's refined fructose that should be avoided.

In conclusion, I am saying that you should eat slow-release carbs and enjoy them. Just make sure you do so in sensible amounts!

Proteins
–Your Best Friends

■ There is no nutrient that affects fat burning and metabolism as much as protein does. Let me provide you with an example: In a study, thirty-five overweight men went on an eight-week diet. They all ate the same number of calories, but the number of proteins varied. The control group lost an average of 12 lb (5.5 kg) while the group that ate more proteins lost an average of 18 lb (8.3 kg) (140).

In essence, protein has five effects. First, it satiates hunger more than any other nutrient per kcal. Secondly, protein contains nitrogen, a substance that is released when the protein is broken down and converted; this process takes energy. Realistically, this means that 25-30 percent of the protein's energy content is lost during this conversion.

Thirdly, protein stimulates the release of the hormone *glucagon*, which releases fats from fat cells and enables more effective fat burning. You therefore burn more fat when you exercise or move, but you also burn fat while at rest. Studies show that increasing your intake from 15 percent of calories from protein (around the same as the average intake per person in Sweden today) up to 30 percent increases fat burning and reduces body fat (115).

The fourth effect is that protein delays the emptying of the stomach; therefore, a meal rich in proteins provides a feeling of fullness that lasts for longer and also allows for a steadier blood-sugar curve. A more balanced blood sugar means less insulin, which has a direct effect on burning fat.

Finally, protein preserves muscle mass. When you diet, you consume fewer calories than you expend, which means you lose fat and muscle at the same time. Due to protein's ability to preserve muscle, the loss of muscle is reduced when the protein intake is high (57, 200).

What Is a Good Source of Protein?

Increasingly, research is showing a distinction between different sources of protein when it comes to their effect on metabolism and energy expenditure. Protein derived from animal sources such as meat, eggs, milk, poultry, fish, and shellfish contain all the essential amino acids—building blocks that the body itself is unable to produce. Animal proteins seem to give a greater increase in energy expenditure than protein derived from vegetarian sources, which are "incomplete" in terms of the essential amino acids (39).

Vegetarian protein sources—beans, nuts, seeds, lentils, peas, salad, vegetables, grains, etc.—contain lots of fiber and anti-nutrients, which reduce the breakdown of protein. Essentially only 80-90 percent of vegetarian protein sources are broken down, meaning you need to eat more to get the same effect on the body as is caused by animal proteins. You may see weight loss, but it's really a result of muscle loss, not fat loss.

Whey and casein are proteins that come from milk that seem to have a particularly good effect on weight. We'll discuss these more in the chapter on milk. Soy protein (found, for example, in soy milk, tofu, and protein powder) is also a type of protein that is beneficial to weight loss beyond just protein content (102). It's not just that the soybean is the legume that is richest in protein, but the quality of the protein is pretty much complete. Maybe the soybean's good effect is due to the substances that affect the body's hormones—there are a plethora of these in soy. Much points to the fact that soy can maintain the production of thyroid hormone during dieting and calorie restriction. When you eat fewer calories, the levels of thyroid hormone drops, leading to a decrease in metabolism. Soy consumption may counter this.

Every Meal Should Contain Protein

Sometimes you see people eating a banana as a snack or drinking a smoothie while waiting for dinner. There is nothing wrong with this, but you also need some protein, preferably about ½ oz to 1 oz (10-30 g), to stabilize your blood sugar and keep you feeling full. You can have a sandwich with a few extra slices of ham, or mix protein powder in your smoothie, or you can even resort to what I call an "essential protein." These are easy and complete sources of protein that can be kept in the refrigerator and quickly grabbed to make a complete snack.

Good examples of "essential proteins" are boiled eggs, roast beef, cooked/tinned soybeans, grilled chicken (e.g. chicken drumsticks), canned fish (e.g. tuna, mackerel, or sardines), cottage cheese, quark, homemade meat patties, and poached salmon. I nearly always boil a few extra eggs to keep in the fridge for a few days. When at the grocery store, I'll often buy chicken drumsticks, but I always remove the skin before eating because grilling the drumsticks forms carcinogenic substances in the skin.

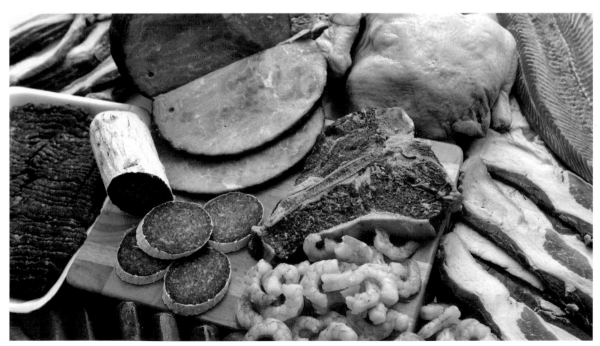

Coconut
–And Other Saturated Fats

■ Saturated fats have long been a hot topic, and they've been accused of having a negative effect on our health, especially when it comes to heart disease, type 2 diabetes, and some forms of cancer. Lately, some have suggested that saturated fat is not as bad as it seems. So, who is right?

The problem is that saturated fats get confused with each other. There are actually a large number of saturated fats that all have different effects on your body. The first mistake researchers in the '60s and '70s made was to compare "hard" (saturated) fats and "soft" (unsaturated) fats and assume that all hard fats were bad and all soft good. This is an incredible generalization. Under the heading "hard fat," not only butter and margarine, but even the dreaded trans fats (which today we know are bad for our health) could be found lurking. In the '80s and '90s, it became evident that trans fats were in a class of their own when it came to being bad, and they were excluded from various studies. However, the remaining natural fats still had such varying effects on our bodies that even lumping these together and picking out an average was not scientifically correct. We

need to distinguish between *short chain* (SCT), *medium chain* (MCT), and *long chain* (LCT) saturated fats, all of which have completely different effects.

Let's Start at the Beginning

In order to understand why saturated fats have so many different effects, we need to start at the beginning. Fat consists of fatty acids, which are a sort of chain of carbon atoms. Most fatty acids have 16 carbon atoms or more; the more carbon atoms, the more soluble the fatty acid. The number of carbon atoms in fatty acids can vary from two to twenty-four, which means that there is a vast difference between how soluble they are. The shortest can be classed as being completely water soluble and not thriving with other fats. Compare water and cooking oil—"water soluble" versus "fat soluble"—they will create two distinct layers if you try to mix them in a glass.

Saturated fatty acids can be divided into three groups depending on how long they are. SCT stands for Short Chain Triglycerides and have two or four carbon atoms. These are the closest to being water soluble, whereas

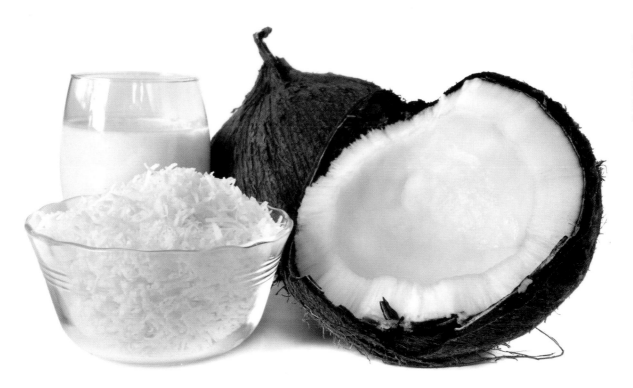

the next group, known as MCT (Medium Chain Triglycerides) have some fat soluble properties but are mainly water soluble. They have six, eight, or ten carbon atoms. The longest are called LCT (Long Chain Triglycerides) and have twelve, fourteen, sixteen, eighteen, twenty, twenty-two, or even twenty-four carbon atoms. There is some variation when it comes to which group the fatty acids are deemed to belong; (those with twelve carbon atoms are sometimes listed as MCT).

Because they are all saturated, they keep well when it comes to heating and storage. It's the unsaturated fats that can oxidize and become damaging. Because coconut fat has a very high content of saturated fats, it's very stable and best to use when frying, deep frying, or other types of cooking that require high temperatures. You will shortly be reading about the health benefits of coconut fat. Olive oil, sunflower oil, rapeseed oil, and similar oils are a lot more sensitive. Butter can be described as something in between that is all right to use when frying at medium to high temperatures. Saturated fats can also be found in many foods that have a long shelf life, such as aged cheese or ham, and they can be stored for many years without turning rancid.

SCT and MCT Act Differently

SCT and MCT have, thanks to their water-soluble properties, a slightly different route through the body compared with long chain fatty acids. SCT and MCT are partially absorbed in the stomach, and the rest is quickly absorbed in the small intestine because they do not require bile to digest. After this, SCT and MCT travel to the liver, where they are used as fuel. The upshot is that the liver gets the energy it needs and heat is released during metabolism. Higher temperatures suppress the appetite, making you stop eating. That which doesn't remain in the liver is released into the blood stream, the muscles, and the mitochondria, where they are able to be burned off and are converted to movement—a walk in the country, for example, or a cleaning session at home.

Very little of the SCT and MCT go to fat cells, in contrast to the long chain fatty acids that are nearly always sent directly to the fat cells to be stored. It's not until some time has passed that they are released and can enter the muscles to be metabolized.

SCT and MCT Don't Need Carnitine

The last step before fat can be metabolized is absorption by the mitochondria—the cells' power station—and this is what limits how much fat can be metabolized. Simply put, we can burn a certain number of ounces of long-chained fat per minute and any energy that the body requires above this has to come from other energy sources. The main source is carbohydrates, but even protein can be used as an energy source. How much long-chained fat can be absorbed and metabolized by the mitochondria depends on the individual. Fitness level is important, and the better aerobic capacity you have, the better the fat burning is. Consuming long-chained fat also increases transport into the mitochondria, but only up to a certain level. If more than 50 percent of your caloric intake comes from fat, the higher the risk that the mitochondria can't actually absorb all of it. Better fitness, therefore, equals a more smoothly running power station.

The limitation is *carnitine*, an amino acid found in the membrane of the mitochondria that lets the long-chained fatty acids in. Without carnitine, LCT can't get metabolized properly. SCT and MCT are able to flow straight into the mitochondria without any need for carnitine. This means that they are much easier for the body to metabolize, and energy-wise, they can be described as something between fast-burning carbohydrates and slow-burning fat. This means that coconut is better for burning fat than most other fats.

Where are SCT and MCT Found?

SCT and MCT can be found in a variety of foods such as coconut, palm kernel oil, and fats from dairy products (for example milk, yogurt, butter, cheese, and cottage cheese). Even breast milk contains SCT and MCT, which shows how important these fats have been to mankind throughout our evolution.

The most pronounced source is coconut, which has no less than 60-70 percent of its fat in the form of SCT and MCT (which is why coconut is the most researched). Fats from dairy contain around 25 percent SCT and MCT, but they also have a high amount of long-chained fatty acids:

around 35 percent. This is why dairy fats are acceptable, within reason, but they should not be over-consumed, as the fat-building properties from LCT will then take over. Read more about LCT in the next shortcut.

Research Results

› A Brazilian study looked at the effect of 1 fl oz (30 ml) coconut oil versus the same amount of soybean oil. The test subjects were forty women aged 20–40 years, who consumed the same diet with an energy deficiency while taking a fifty-minute walk each day. The study continued for twelve weeks. All participants lost weight, but those who received the coconut oil were the only ones to reduce their waist measurements (80).

› A Canadian study of twenty healthy women aged 19–26 years showed that coconut oil could increase the metabolism of LCT. Coconut oil also enabled their bodies to use more LCT as fuel, which is important information because coconut fat also contains LCT (81).

› I seldom reference animal studies, but this one is fascinating and can explain why coconut is so beneficial to weight. Rats who received coconut fat produced more UCP1, a protein found in the so called "brown fat." UCP1 is responsible for brown fat converting fat to heat, or fuel for the fire. If the same applies to humans, it is very exciting indeed (82).

› Is MCT even better for your weight than olive oil? We know that olive oil beats most fat sources when it comes to losing weight, but this sixteen-week study of forty-nine overweight men showed that MCT is actually better. The test subjects got around ¾ oz (20 g) of either olive oil or MCT each day. Both the subcutaneous fat and belly fat were reduced in the group that were given MCT, meaning that they lost around 3 lb (1.5 kg) more than the olive oil group (83).

› A Chinese study of forty slightly overweight type 2 diabetics showed consuming about ½ oz (18 g) MCT a day over ninety days caused a reduction in weight and better sensitivity to insulin compared to an equal amount of corn oil (84).

- A Canadian study examined the MCT fat's effect on burning fat. Nineteen healthy men with a normal weight were given either MCT or olive oil over the course of four weeks. It was evident that the metabolism and fat burn tended to increase with the MCT group, and when the study was complete, they had lost on average 2.2 lb (1 kg). The olive oil group had only lost around 1.3 lb (0.6 kg) (85).

- In another study of overweight men, it was shown that twenty-eight days of taking either MCT or olive oil made a difference. Those who received MCT lost on average 1.5 lb (0.7 kg) whereas the others did not lose any weight (86).

- The same researchers also showed that MCT increased metabolism in overweight women as opposed to fat from hamburger meat, when they were given it over a course of four weeks. They were given 40 percent of calories from fat of which 75 percent was made up of the fats that were to be studied. The MCT group used 0.95 kcal/minute and 0.080 g fat/min as opposed to 0.90 kcal/min and 0.075 g fat/minute for those given tallow fat (87).

- A Japanese study looked at the effect of MCT versus LCT on seventy-eight healthy men and women of average weight over twelve weeks. They ate around 2,250 kcal/day and around 2 oz (60 g) fat, which is equivalent to 24 percent of calories from fat. Those with a BMI over 23 lost an average of 8 ½ lb (3.86 kg) with MCT while those eating LCT lost 6 lb (2.75 kg) (88).

- In one study, the researchers wanted to measure if there was a difference in thermogenesis after a meal consisting of ½ oz (14 g) rapeseed oil or the equivalent of an oil containing 12 percent MCT. Even at the low levels of MCT, it was evident that thermogenesis was higher up to six hours after a meal with MCT (111).

Eating Coconut?

Because coconut oil is so good for your health and weight and is very heat stable, I would like to bring it into the spotlight. If you plan to fry, wok, or deep-fry anything, coconut oil is perfect, and it works just as well with the basic types that can be found in your local store. Of course, it is a refined fat, which means you lose some antioxidants, but considering the high number of saturated fats in coconut, there are practically no trans fats when it's refined. When, for example, rapeseed oil is refined and made odorless and colorless, around ½ to 2 percent trans fats are formed, which does not sound very good. If you really want the most natural fat, there is cold-pressed coconut fat in health food stores, but it's fairly expensive and does taste of coconut, which isn't always suitable. If you want one that doesn't taste of coconut, there is an organic, cold pressed option; it is, however, refined. Personally, I use refined coconut oil for frying, and if you plan to make popcorn at home, it's the obvious choice.

Eat coconut fresh, shredded, or grated. Fresh coconut is delicious and is great for snacking or as a part of your breakfast. It's just a question of cracking the nut and getting to the meat, but it's well worth the effort. And in my opinion, few raw foods taste this delicious! Grated coconut is perfect for baking with, adding to fruit salads, and combining with muesli, to name a few. Coconut milk is also a fantastic ingredient in different recipes, and stews, soups, sauces, and oven baked foods all benefit from a dash of it.

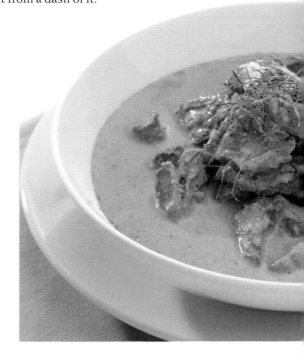

Go Easy on the Bacon

–Saturated Fats You Should Avoid

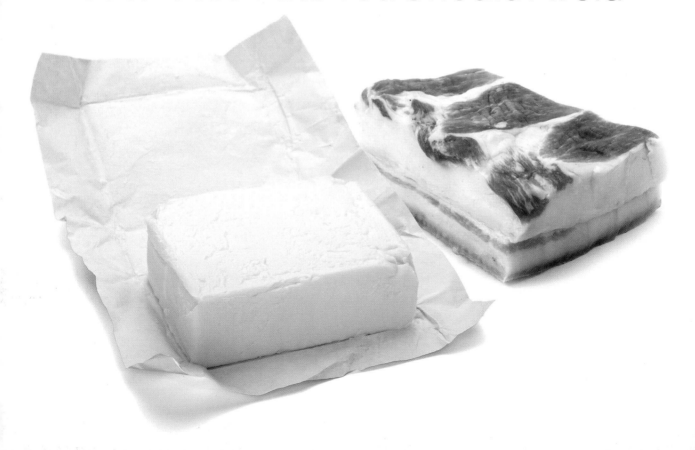

■ Now let's discuss the saturated fats known as LCT—the long-chained fats that can be found in copious amounts in fatty animal products, such as sausages, bacon, fatty meat, and lard. Even fats in dairy have about 35 percent LCT in them, but these also contain a number of other fats that balance out LCT's negative effects. Physiologically, LCTs are the best fats in terms of being stored by the body for later use. They are very fat soluble and can, therefore, thrive in the fat cells (unlike SCT and MCT); in addition, they don't turn rancid. This means LCTs can be stored for longer periods, a trick human bodies have learned through evolution, and there are a host of mechanisms that make long-chained saturated fats affect weight gain. First and foremost, LCTs lower your sensitivity to insulin (103), which means that more insulin is required to regulate your blood sugar (to unlock the cells, so that blood sugar is absorbed). Insulin is also a hormone that enables the fat cells to absorb fats—so, more insulin makes us fatter!

It takes a while before sensitivity to insulin deteriorates, but the fact is that a combination of fats at each meal can have an effect. A meal with a large number of saturated fats causes higher insulin and blood sugar levels than a meal with a large number of unsaturated fats (104, 107). As soon as the consumption of saturated fats increases, energy expenditure and fat burning seem to decrease. In fact, overweight children tend to have more saturated fats in their belly fat than what is present in their food (105). Frightening, isn't it?

The Wrong Saturated Fats Are Difficult to Digest

It seems that the long-chained saturated fats are harder to metabolize in the muscles than monounsaturated or polyunsaturated fats. Unsaturated fats exist in two forms—monounsaturated and polyunsaturated—and can be found in abundance in olive oil, avocado, rapeseed oil, and fish. You can read more about unsaturated fats later on in this book. Studies show that long-chained saturated fats are harder for the body to burn during exercise than unsaturated fats (106). This is important both for individuals who wish to lose weight and those wanting to increase endurance.

Research Results

Here is a review of what happens if you eat too many long-chained saturated fats. Please note that some of the studies do not take into account what sort of saturated fat has been consumed (SCT, MCT, or LCT), and that the fattening properties of LCT would become clearer if these were isolated.

› An Australian study examined what happens to weight in overweight men who either ate a lot of saturated fats or predominantly monounsaturated fats. They had food served to them over the course of four weeks; the only difference was that one group got 24 percent of calories from saturated fat, while the other group got 11 percent. In total, they ate 40 percent of calories from fat, and the rest was unsaturated fats with an emphasis on monounsaturated fats. When the trial period was over, those who ate the least saturated fats lost 4 ½ lb (2.1 kg) more weight and a total of 5 ¾ lb (2.6 kg) more pure fat than those who ate a lot of saturated fats (108).

› In an American study of older individuals, there were two factors that determined constitution: Those who moved the most and ate less saturated fat had the least body fat and more muscle mass (109).

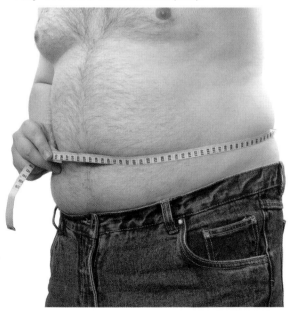

- In a Spanish study, scientists let the subjects (twenty-nine healthy men aged 18-30 years) eat three portions with the same number of calories, but different combinations of fat. After receiving fat from either mainly walnuts (polyunsaturated and monounsaturated), olive oil (monounsaturated), or dairy products (saturated), their production of heat (thermogenesis) was measured over a period of five hours. The walnut group had a 28 percent higher rate of thermogenesis than the dairy group, and the olive oil group's thermogenesis rate was 23 percent higher than that of the dairy group. I am sure that had they used cured meats rather than dairy products, the effect would have been greater (110).

- Two groups of males aged 25-48 years ate a diet with 46 percent calories from fat for fourteen days. The difference between the two groups was the number of saturated fats. The group that ate less saturated fat had a P/S ratio of 1.67, while those who ate a lot of saturated fats had a P/S ratio of 0.19. The P/S ratio is simply the amount of polyunsaturated fats divided by the amount of saturated fats calculated by grams. After fourteen days, the basal metabolic rate was 0.17 kj higher per minute for those who ate some saturated fat *before* breakfast. Those who ate some saturated fat *after* breakfast had 0.29 kj/minute higher thermogenesis over the next four hours. It might sound like a small difference, but over the course of a year, this adds up to an energy quantity of 6 ½ lb (3 kg), if you take into account the increased basal energy expenditure (112).

- Another study measured how different fats directly affect fat burning. The subjects ate either a high P/S ratio (a lot of polyunsaturated fats and a little saturated) or a low one. The trial lasted for more than a week, and you could see that the diet with a little saturated fat meant a lower rate of fat burning. On average, subjects burned 0.059 g fat/minute as opposed to 0.074 g fat/minute for those who ate more unsaturated fats. It might not sound like a lot, but remember that this difference can remain day in, day out, week in, week out (114).

- In a Spanish study, a group of men with high cholesterol aged 18-63 years replaced part of the saturated fats in their diet with olive oil for twenty-eight days. They were not eating fewer calories, just better fats (38 percent of calories). The results showed that their body fat was reduced from an average of 51.37 lb (23.3 kg) to 45.86 lb (20.8 kg), while their muscle mass increased. Even those who ate a high amount of carbs (57 percent of calories) improved their body constitution compared to when they ate a large quantity of long-chained saturated fat (116).

- We know that long-chained saturated fats can reduce sensitivity to insulin, which is related to an increase in belly fat. A typical apple-shaped body is usually the result of a lowered sensitivity to insulin. In a study of diabetics, five overweight but otherwise healthy subjects and six average weight and healthy subjects ate either a lot of saturated fat or a lot of polyunsaturated fat for a course of five weeks. Sensitivity to insulin increased, and subcutaneous fat around the stomach was reduced amongst those who ate more polyunsaturated fats (117).

- In a study of older women with some abdominal fat, the effects of olive oil were compared to cream. When measured five hours after a meal, olive oil was shown to better increase fat burning. At the same time, the meal-induced thermogenesis was increased for the olive oil group (118).

- One of the largest studies in this area used 41,518 female nurses aged 41-68 years who varied in weight. The study showed that animal fats and trans fats were those that were most linked to weight gain. Amongst overweight subjects, trans fats had a significant effect on weight gain. For every percent of fat intake represented by trans fats, the women gained about 2 ½ lb (1.2 kg). If 10 percent of the energy intake came from trans fats, that would amount to about a around 26 ½ lb (12 kg) weight gain. Monounsaturated and polyunsaturated fats did not increase the risk for weight gain (163).

Products to Avoid if You Want to Burn Fat:

- **Bacon**
- **Pork belly**
- **Fatty sausages**
- **Minced pork**
- **Tallow**
- **Too many fatty dairy products (cream, butter, cheese)**

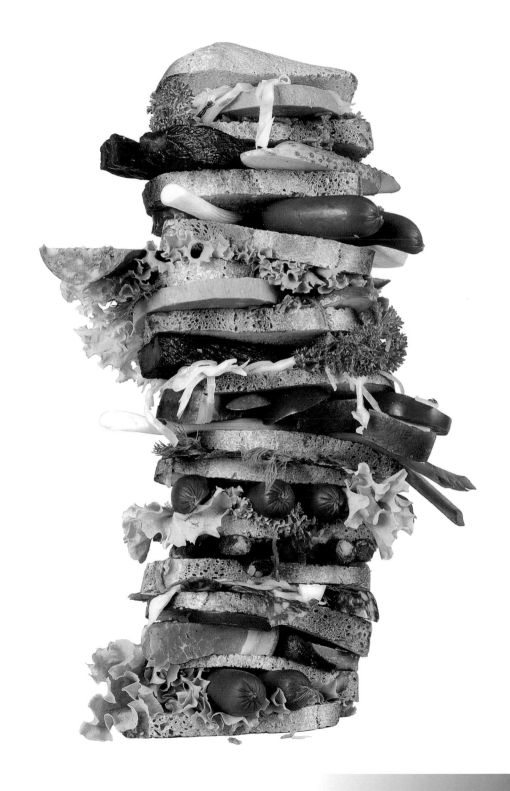

Essential Unsaturated Fats
–Get the Right Balance

Poly- and monounsaturated fats belong to the larger category of unsaturated fats. Polyunsaturated fat is a relatively large group of fats and includes, among others, omega-3 fats whose fat burning properties you can read about in the fish shortcut on page 32. Other polyunsaturated fats include omega-6 fatty acids, such as linoleic acid and GLA. Linoleic acid is the most common polyunsaturated fatty acid and is an "essential fatty acid"; this means that it is a part of our diet vital to our survival. The richest sources of omega-6 fatty acids are vegetable oils such as corn, soybean, peanut, grape seed, and thistle oils. But omega-6 fatty acids can also be found in nearly all other sources of fat. It's almost impossible to be deficient in omega-6 fatty acids as long as you consume a normal amount of fat.

Omega-6 Burns Fat

Linoleic acid is a polyunsaturated fatty acid and is, as mentioned earlier, sensitive to oxidation. This means it can turn rancid and become dangerous to your health;

for example, it can increase the risk of cancer, lower your cell functions, cause inflammations, etc. This is why the body wants to protect itself against omega-6 fatty acids by burning them off before they become dangerous; so, the more omega-6 you consume, the higher the fat burning. Omega-6 acts as an inhibitor to the storage of fat in two ways: It inhibits the conversion of carbohydrates and protein into fat (205)–something that can otherwise occur both in the fat cells and liver–And, secondly, fatty acids with a high grade of unsaturation (omega-6, for example) are released more easily from the fat cells than other fats (206).

In conclusion, you can say that omega-6 would be damaging if the body did not burn it off, but the body has clearly found a clever solution to the problem. In addition, it's important to eat the right amount of omega-3 (see next page) to get the perfect balance for your body.

We know that omega-6 fatty acids increase fat burning more than most other fatty acids, but before

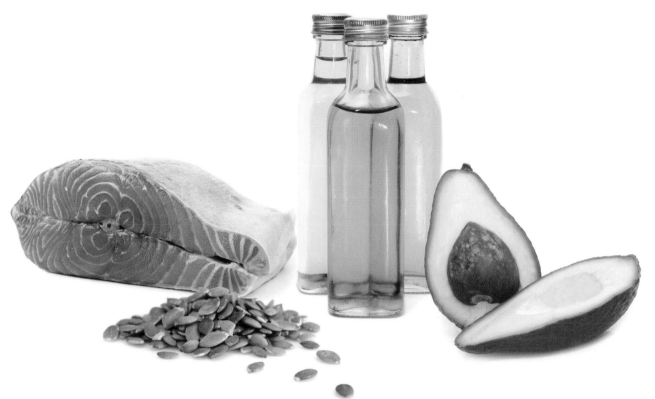

you order the catch of the day, consider this: Omega-3 and omega-6 compete with each other in the body to become *eicosanoids*—fast-acting molecules that affect blood vessels, inflammations, and the blood's ability to coagulate, among other things. If you eat the same amount of omega-3 and omega-6, your body will be in balance and everything will work properly; however, if you eat too much omega-6, the blood vessels will contract a little too much, leading to high blood pressure and low oxygen levels in the blood. At the same time, inflammatory processes can become too active, causing pain and an increase in cell division, which can lead to cancer and autoimmune diseases.

If you eat too much omega-3 and not enough omega-6, you'll get the opposite: decreased coagulation of the blood and an increased risk of severe bleeding. So, it's important to eat a lot of omega-3 and balance it with a good quantity of omega-6. It seems that omega-6 does not have any negative effects so long as we also get enough omega-3, so even if it feels complicated, the result is quite simple.

Eat fatty fish (mackerel, salmon, Baltic herring, etc.) three times a week and use a lot of vegetable fat when cooking—olive oil, rapeseed oil, avocado oil, and nut oils are especially good (monounsaturated fats). Seeds are a good source of omega-6 because they contain so many other nutrients, such as protein, antioxidants, fiber, and so on. If you don't like to eat fatty fish, it's just as beneficial to eat double the amount of lean fish or shellfish; even mussels, shrimp, and crab contain omega-3. The only thing I absolutely do not recommend is increasing your intake of omega-6 without balancing it with omega-3 because that will increase the risk of inflammation and health problems. On the other hand, a balanced diet of omega-6 and omega-3 can lead you to the best shape of your life!

Dairy Products

–Can Make You Thin

Dairy products such as milk, yogurt, sour milk, cottage cheese, quark, and protein powders with casein, whey, or milk certainly have their place in a book about burning fat. Studies show that if you eat these products regularly, you can increase your ability to burn fat while sparing your muscle mass. It's hard to point out just what it is that makes dairy products so suited to building a better body. There are several components to dairy products that can contribute to this effect (95), and you can read about some of these under their own headings in this book. One is the short- and medium-chained fatty acids (SCT and MCT) that make up about a quarter of the fats in dairy products. Another is CLA (see the shortcut on this on page 97), which appears in varying degrees in different products, and a third component is calcium, which we all know contributes to weight loss. In dairy products, the effects of these components seem to be greater than when they appear in products on their own, and this can partly be explained by the protein in milk. Around 80 percent of milk's protein is casein and 20 percent is whey, and both of these types of protein are known to have positive effects on weight. Many dairy products are even good sources of vitamin D. A review of the studies available has shown that the calcium in milk lowers pH levels in the small intestine and inhibits the absorption of fat. A dose of 1200 mg (the amount of calcium in 1 ¾ pints [1 liter] of milk) extra calcium per day (above normal consumption) can, according to these studies, cause about 0.18 ounces (5 grams) of fat loss per day (96). It might not sound like much, but this is equivalent to forty-five calories, and over a year this adds up to about 16,000 kcal—the energy amount in roughly 4 ½ lb (2 kg) of body fat.

What Are the "Right" Dairy Products?

When it comes to the effect on fat burning, there is a lot of variation between dairy products, and you shouldn't generalize by saying that all dairy based products can be freely consumed. Products such as butter, cream, high-fat cheeses, crème fraîche, and sour cream are not beneficial to your weight. Of course, they have some fat that is okay for you (SCT and MCT), but they don't contain enough protein or calcium (the main reasons why dairy products are included in this book).

Dairy products that are really good for burning fat are curds (quark), cottage cheese, lean cheeses, low-fat milk, and yogurt/sour milk. Of course, these should be the sugar-free varieties because sugar vastly inhibits the burning of fat.

That dairy products are so varied in their makeup is the reason why some studies do not show any effects, while some even demonstrate that "dairy products" make you gain weight (97). In these instances, they are talking about products that are high in fat and low in protein and that quickly give you an excess of energy.

Research Results

Milk protein supplements are what often hides in the tins of protein found in health food shops, grocery stores, and online. Generally the protein is mixed with different forms of carbohydrate sources.

> A study of overweight American police officers showed that the results of a twelve-week diet (they ate 80 percent of their energy expenditure) varied depending on whether they took supplements or not. They were divided into three groups that took either casein, whey, or no supplement at all. The supplements gave 1.5 g protein per kg per day. The average loss of fat was 5 ½ lb (2.5 kg) in all groups, but those who received casein increased their muscle mass by nearly 9 lb (4 kg). Those receiving whey had to make do with a

2.2 lb (2 kg) gain in muscle mass, so in this little study it seems that casein caused the best change to the body's constitution (92).

> Another study shows that both casein and whey are equally good in maintaining the weight of a person who has lost weight on a diet (93).

> Even whey has a good effect on the body, especially when it comes to exercise. In this study, whey beat out casein when it came to reducing body fat and increasing muscle mass. Thirteen male body builders worked out intensely over a ten-week period. They were given 1.5 g whey or casein per kg per day. The whey group increased by a whole 11 lb (5 kg) of muscle mass, while the casein group only gained 1.75 lb (.8 kg) muscle. When it came to fat, the whey group decreased by 3.3 lb (1.5 kg), while the group that took casein, on average, lost nothing. So as you can see, research illustrates both sides, and the only thing I can promise you is that, after exercise, both casein and whey build muscle and can contribute to lowering body fat (94).

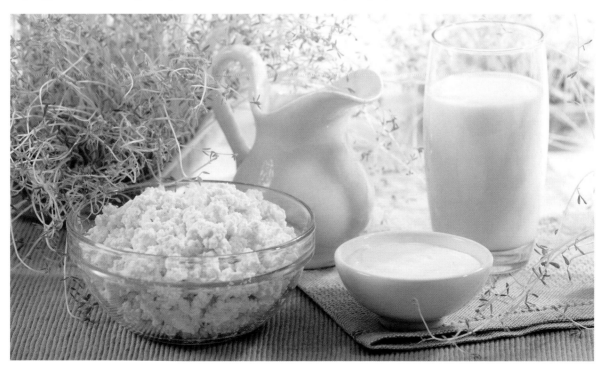

Fish

–Oh, the Super Fats

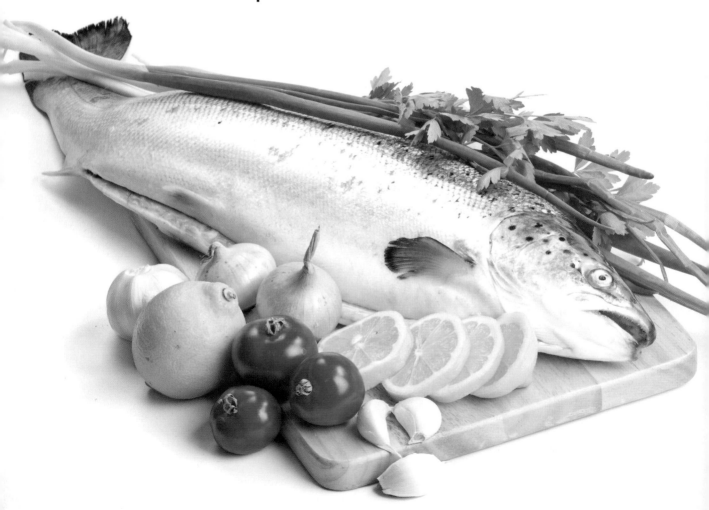

Many people feel that they keep trim and feel better when they eat a lot of fish, shellfish, and other foods from the sea. My belief is that you shouldn't put too much emphasis on subjective views—always have some science to back up your claims.

So, what about seafood? Does it increase fat burning, and does it help keep your weight steady? Yes, when you assess all the research, it is very clear that this is the case. The reasons are numerous, and I would like to start by going through the available theories and then describing what happens when you eat fish.

Omega-3: Your Metabolizing Fat

Omega-3 fatty acids from the sea are very special. We know they do a lot of good for our health, but these are also the fats that are easily destroyed by warmth and oxygen. Omega-3 fatty acids can oxidize, and when this occurs in the body, it increases the risk of inflammation and serious illnesses like heart disease, type 2 diabetes, and many forms of cancer. So, omega-3 fatty acids don't store very easily in your fat cells; on the contrary, it seems that when you consume omega-3, your body becomes aware that there is fat that can easily become rancid, and that the burning of fat has to increase to ensure that your health does not deteriorate.

Omega-3 for Insulin Sensitivity

As you may remember, we said earlier that a healthy sensitivity to insulin leads to a decreased need it; this reduces the amount of stored fat and increases fat burning. So, I ought to tell you that omega-3 fats from fish increase your sensitivity to insulin (137). The reason for this is because fat from fish is very runny. You can imagine what it must be like inside a fish living in the cold water; if its fats were not this runny, the fish would become as stiff as a fish stick and sink straight to the bottom! When you eat fish fats, they blend into your cell membranes and make them soft. When insulin binds to the receptors on the cell's surface, a signal goes through the membrane and into the cell. If you have a high amount of hard fats in the cell membrane—caused by eating too many long-chained saturated fats (sausages, bacon, and fatty pork, to name a few), the signals are inhibited and your sensitivity to insulin decreases. If instead you

have soft fats making the cell membrane soft, it becomes easier for the signal from the insulin receptor to enter the cell, and sensitivity to insulin improves. Therefore, if you eat fish regularly, not only will you get a flatter stomach, but you will also protect yourself against type 2 diabetes.

Research Results

> In one study, 126 people were divided into three groups and followed a diet with 30 percent less energy consumption over eight weeks. All the subjects had the same energy intake and were given the same amount of fat, proteins, and carbohydrates. The only thing that separated the groups was the amount of cod consumed. The control group did not eat any cod at all, group one received 5.3 oz (150 g) of cod three times a week, and group two ate 5.3 oz (150 g) of cod five times a week. All of the subjects lost weight, but group two lost 3.75 lb (1.7 kg) more than the control. Even group one lost more than the control group, and the effect seemed to be related to the cod (138).

> Another study had 324 women and men aged 20–40 years follow a diet that was identical apart from the seafood content. The control group received no fish, fish oil, or shellfish at all. In the eight-week study, the other three groups ate either three portions of 5.3 oz (150 g) of cod a week, three portions of 5.3 oz (150 g) of salmon a week, or the recommended daily dose of fish oil. All three groups that ate seafood lost about 4 ½ lb (2 kg) more that the control during the study, although the results were more significant for men than for women (139).

> Even when you eat a breakfast that is low in carbs, fish is a smart choice. In this study, people who were slightly overweight ate a diet low in carbs for four weeks; the fat content of their diet came from either mainly red meat (group one) or mainly fish, shell fish, and poultry (group two). Group one lost an average of 11.6 lb (5.26 kg), while group two lost an average of 12.65 lb (5.74 kg) despite the energy intake being identical between the two groups. In addition, in group two the triglycerids in the blood were demonstrated to be lowered, which protects against heart disease (141).

> Omega-3 can also make us feel fuller. One study measured the feelings of fullness during a diet, and those who ate more than 1300 mg omega-3 per day felt an increased feeling of fullness immediately after the meal and for up to two hours afterwards than those who ate less than 260 mg omega-3 per day (142).

Breakfast
–For Maximum Metabolism

"Eat breakfast like a king, lunch like a prince, and dinner like a pauper." Fitness icon Dolph Lundgren quoted this old adage in a television interview I was watching, and there's a lot to be said for this mantra. When you wake up, your blood sugar is low, and depleted hormones circulate in the blood. If you go too long on an empty stomach, your muscle mass will begin to break down. This is why breakfast is so important! By eating a healthy meal when you wake up, you halt this process and build up energy reserves, so that you can better manage until lunch. This means that your body will have an easier time handling blood sugar, and you use blood sugar more easily during your waking hours. In the chapter on morning exercise (see page 112), you'll read that it's okay to wait for up to one and a half hours after first waking without eating any breakfast, but if you stave off for any longer than this, things starts to get out of control. The metabolizing processes take over, and both your immune system and muscle mass are negatively affected. Your blood sugar sinks so much that you will forget your good

eating habits, and your reptilian brain takes over and decides—or rather screams at you—what you should eat. The result is white bread rolls with marmalade, sugary yogurts, Nutella, and any other rubbish that tastes delicious. Those who don't eat breakfast tend to consume more calories once the day is over compared with those who do eat their breakfast. So, the lesson from this is skipping: Skipping breakfast can actually make you fat.

Breakfast for Children

An interesting article on weight collated a number of scientific studies of nearly 60,000 children that examined the weight of children who either ate breakfast or skipped it altogether. Generally, they showed that eating breakfast had a protective effect when it came to the risk of becoming overweight (53).

Another health benefit of breakfast is shown by the fact that the food eaten by breakfast skippers during the day tends to have a lower nutritional value, and the risk

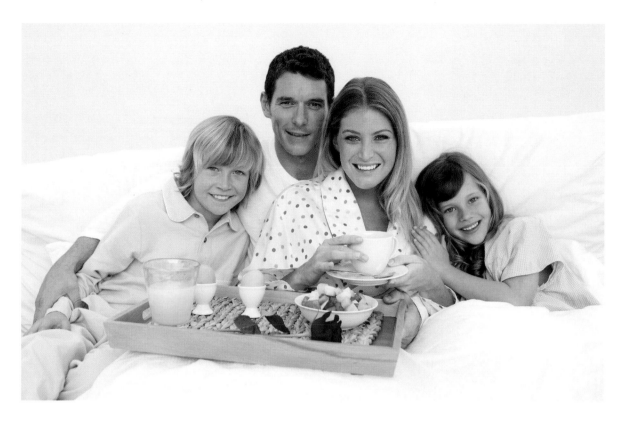

of heart disease and type 2 diabetes seems to increase later in life (54). We also know that children who eat breakfast are better able to concentrate in school and get better grades—so breakfast is important on several levels.

What Sort of Breakfast Should You Eat?

Because people are usually quite conservative when it comes to choice of breakfast—normally eating the same foods day after day—it's important that it be as healthy as possible. As always, the basic principles are a mix of fats (good quality fats), protein, and low glycemic index carbs. With this, you should have no problems lasting until lunchtime, and your concentration will be on top all morning. To really eat a breakfast that keeps the metabolism going, it's important to take in a good number of carbs that have a low GI. Around 33 percent of the energy should come from carbs (see the iso diet).

One study showed that low GI and the right amount of carbs caused a better rate of fat burning and higher metabolism than the same caloric intake in the form of high GI and lots of carbs (55). The increase in metabolism was due to the fact that thermogenesis (heat production) rose after breakfast.

Examples of a Good Breakfast

- Omelet and fruit salad
- Oat porridge with milk and a boiled egg
- Natural yogurt with unsweetened muesli and a handful of nuts
- Unsweetened whole grain bread with mackerel in tomato sauce
- A selection of fruits and two boiled eggs
- Three eggs over easy and thawed berries with some runny honey
- Smoothie with yogurt, flax seeds, and berries

Evening Snacks
–Take It Easy

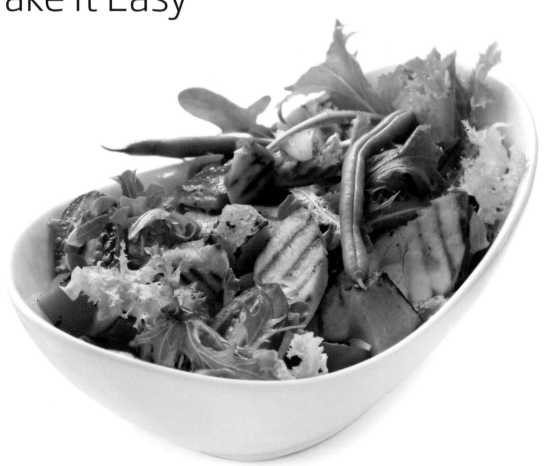

■ Are you the kind of person who eats food late at night? Then you need to read this chapter carefully and learn to get away from nighttime snacking.

First, it's never great to eat large amounts of calories late at night before going to bed because your energy expenditure is greatly reduced. Over the coming hours, your body simply won't need the food you're eating, and the consequences are obvious: The excess will get stored as fat. When you're awake and moving, your energy expenditure is roughly double that of when you are asleep. In addition, your muscles are much hungrier for blood sugar when you're awake. When you use your muscles, they require energy, which means that the blood sugar that is released after, breakfast, for example, enters the muscles more quickly and is never given the chance to reach alarming levels. If you eat the same food just before bedtime, it won't be as effectively absorbed into your resting muscles causing your blood sugar to become significantly higher. This isn't good for your health and will lead to the production of more insulin—once again resulting in higher fat storage.

Secondly, research shows that a high insulin level at night automatically leads to a lower level of growth hormone, and this hormone is vital to burning fat.

Keep Your Evening Snack Low in Carbs

If, like most people, you sleep at night and are awake during the day, it's smart to make the last meal of the day contain relatively few carbs. The fewer hours between the last meal of the day and bedtime, the more important this becomes. The main reason is that your muscles are inactive during the night and the body goes into a state of relaxation. This means that the last meal of the day tends to raise the blood sugar more than earlier meals, even if they are nutritionally identical. High blood sugar causes damage in terms of AGE (advanced glycation end products, i.e., products that are formed during glycation), which occurs when the blood sugar reacts with the proteins in the body. In addition to causing inflammation, this advances ageing and increases the risk of heart disease. A night time sandwich à la Dagwood is, therefore, very unhealthy.

Avoid the Nighttime Sandwich!

There is something called "Night Eating Syndrome" (NES), when you regularly get up at night and eat—and it's usually not the healthiest of foods that are consumed. Those who have NES often eat things like cake, chocolate, and biscuits rather than brown rice, salmon, and broccoli. All types of nighttime eating are bad, though, as the body is not designed to accept food at this period, and unhealthy foods make the problem even worse.

Your gut really wants to rest and recuperate at night—something that's a lot easier when there isn't food on its way into the system. For instance, did you know that the inside of the small intestine pretty much gets replaced every two days and that most of this repair happens at night?

If you eat 25 percent or more of your daily caloric intake after dinner, or if you wake up to eat at least three times a week over at least three months, you may be suffering from NES (99). If you belong to this group, you should talk to your doctor because NES can seriously damage your health.

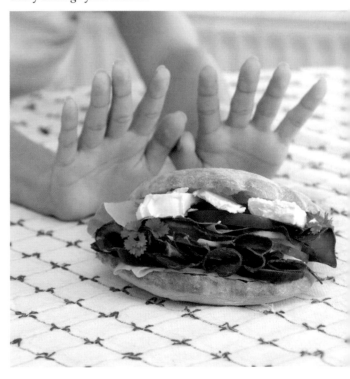

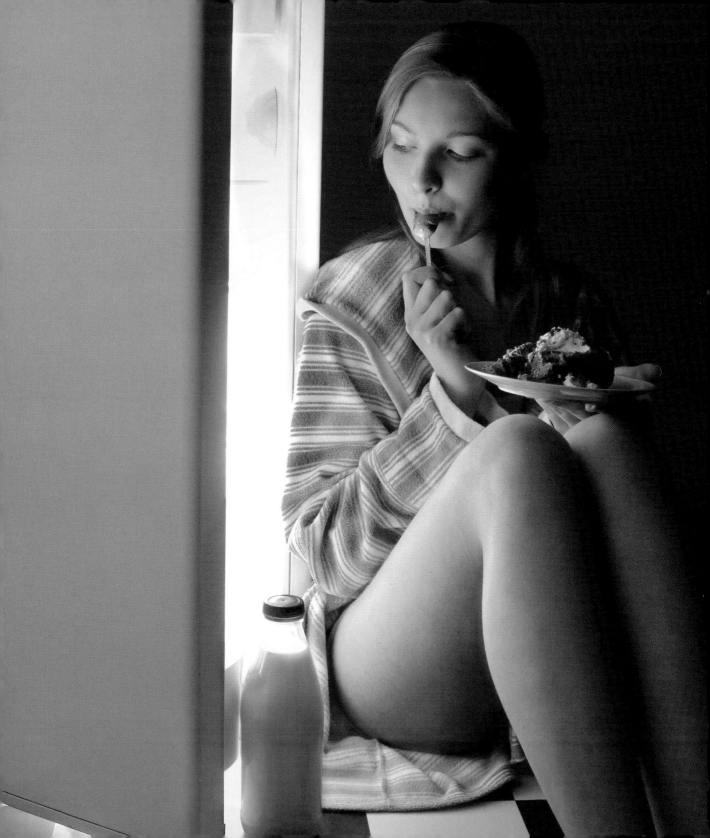

Research Results

> A study examined 375 men and 492 women with respect to how full they got after eating at different times of the day. The subjects registered how much they ate at the following times: 6 AM-9:59 AM, 10 AM-1:59 PM, 2 PM-5:59 PM, 6 PM-9:59 PM, and 10 PM-1:59 AM. The results showed that the more they ate earlier in the day, the fewer calories they needed to be satisfied. Similarly, one can infer that calories that are consumed later in the day do not fill you up as well and can easily lead to weight gain (98).

> Night eating is even worse than a late meal because you break your sleep and consume unnecessary calories. In a Danish study of over 2000 men and women, 9 percent of women and 7.4 percent of men were night eaters. When researchers looked at their weight gain over a six-year period, they saw that the overweight women who ate at night had gained 11.5 lb (5.2 kg) on average. For the men, the trend was not as strong, and women of average weight gained only about 2 lb (0.9 kg) (100).

   Altogether it seems that overweight women are the most vulnerable when it comes to night eating–possibly because of what they eat. A man who gets up at night to eat might not take a piece of cake, but rather a chicken leg, and this is obviously better for your weight.

> An American study of overweight people who went on a diet to lose weight showed that eating at night had a considerably negative effect on the results of the diet. Seventy-six patients were classed as normal or night eaters. The latter category consisted of those who either skipped breakfast (morning anorexia) at least four times a week, ate at least 50 percent of their calorie intake after 7 PM, or had a hard time falling asleep/sleeping at least four nights a week. Night eaters felt worse, were more depressed, had lower self-esteem, and had a reduced appetite earlier in the day. In addition, they only lost on average 9.7 lb (4.4 kg) during the month that the diet took place as compared to an average of 16 lb (7.3 kg) for those who were not night eaters (101).

> Nine young men were given identical meals at three different times: 9 AM, 5 PM, and 1 AM. The interesting thing was that the mealtime-induced thermogenesis was lower the later the mealtime took place. It is, therefore, easier to gain weight by eating late in the day. The opposite holds true as well (119).

Eat Dinner at the Same Location Every Day

Regular dinner habits are surprisingly important because it's easy to overcompensate later in the evening if you haven't had a proper dinner. Then you open yourself up to all the problems that I just described. In addition, it's important to eat your meals at the dinner table and not, for example, while watching TV. Dinner in front of the TV especially makes children fatter (56). Why this occurs is hard to say, but it's possible that you eat more when the TV distracts you from regulating your appetite. Even the simple fact that the whole family is sitting at the table together and eating seems to give some protection against children becoming overweight (58), and there is no reason to believe that adults work any differently.

What Should the Last Meal of the Day Look Like?

Generally it's not good to eat a normal meal less than three hours before going to bed. If you keep this timeframe between food and bed, your blood sugar has time to rise and normalize before sleep, and you won't get the negative effects that raised blood sugar causes. As you get nearer to bedtime, you should consume fewer carbs. A few good examples of food you can eat an hour before bedtime are:

- **A piece of fried chicken breast with cooked broccoli**
- **Tuna salad made with tuna in water, lots of vegetables, and three tablespoons of an olive oil based dressing**
- **9 oz (250 g) cottage cheese, 10 chopped walnuts, and a few blueberries for flavor**
- **1 grilled chicken drumstick and a salad with chopped tomato, red onion, basil, and two tablespoons of an olive oil-based dressing**
- **3 ½ oz (100 g) peeled prawns and one tablespoon aioli**
- **One omelet made with three eggs, and a glass of vegetable juice**
- **3 ½ oz (100 g) cooked green beans, baby spinach, an avocado, and a splash of vinegar**

   These examples raise blood sugar slowly, but leave you satisfied overnight.

Fibers
–Give Fewer Calories

■ The definition of what fiber really is isn't completely clear, but most researchers count indigestible portions of plant food as dietary fibers due to the plant's cell walls, which are rich in cellulose. Opinions on dietary fiber have changed somewhat in recent years, and the fact is that most of what cannot be digested in the stomach and intestine can be counted as dietary fiber. There are soluble and insoluble fibers that have different properties and consistencies. There are even less-researched fibers in products such as milk, but for the most part, we get fiber from vegetables.

There are two factors that best determine the fibers' properties. The first one is viscosity—how much water the fibers absorb or the amount of gelatinous substances they form in the gut. If a type of fiber becomes very gelatinous, it affects the process of emptying the stomach and the absorption of blood sugar in a beneficial way. One example of this is crushed flax seeds; these contribute a number of soluble and gelatinous fibers, and in this way can lower the GI levels of another food that is consumed simultaneously. Baking with flax seed is therefore a good strategy.

The other factor that determines fiber's effect on health and weight is whether it is fermented by bacteria in the gut. If it is, it can contribute to a better intestinal flora and possibly weight loss.

How Do Fibers Work?

There are many studies that show that a high fiber intake contributes to weight loss (169,170). Fibers work whether they are taken as supplements (310, 311) or as part of a fiber-rich meal (308). One important reason for this is that they reduce the absorption of fat and other nutrients; foods rich in fiber have 2-10 percent fewer calories in reality than is stated on the product label. There does seem to be a limit to how many calories can avoid absorption. Long term, this obviously has a big effect on the fat deposits. This is really the kind of food humans are made for; throughout our evolution, our fiber intake has been high, and we have not absorbed the food fully (something we pretty much always do with modern, highly refined food). All types of fibers tend to be filling (312, 313), which obviously contributes to being in better shape. Soluble fibers tend to be more filling than insoluble fibers if you look at the ability to create a feeling of satiety per gram of fiber. Some foods rich in fiber that have been studied and are proven to be particularly filling are oats (both cooked and as grain), quinoa, and buckwheat (314).

The King of Fat-Burning Fibers

There is a form of fiber known as resistant starch, which is classed as the third form of dietary fiber after the soluble and insoluble fibers. We are talking about starch products that are chains of sugars, which are not digested in the small intestine. The cause of their "resistance" is that humans lack the enzymes to digest the starch, and it, therefore, acts as a form of fiber. It exists naturally in potatoes and bananas and is created when prepared foods rich in starch are left to cool down. Cooked rice, pasta, noodles, and especially all cold potatoes naturally produce some resistant starch. Even legumes and many modern types of breads contain resistant starch. White bread with a high fiber content often contains added resistant starch because it is flavorless and does not significantly affect the baking process.

Interestingly, it seems that a daily supplement of resistant starch can increase sensitivity to insulin and reduce the waistline (315). A study showed that when 5.4 percent of carbohydrates were in the form of resistant starch, fat burning increased by 23 percent compared to those who ate the same food but without the resistant starch (316). It's very simple to add resistant starch when making bread or pasta, for example, without altering the taste.

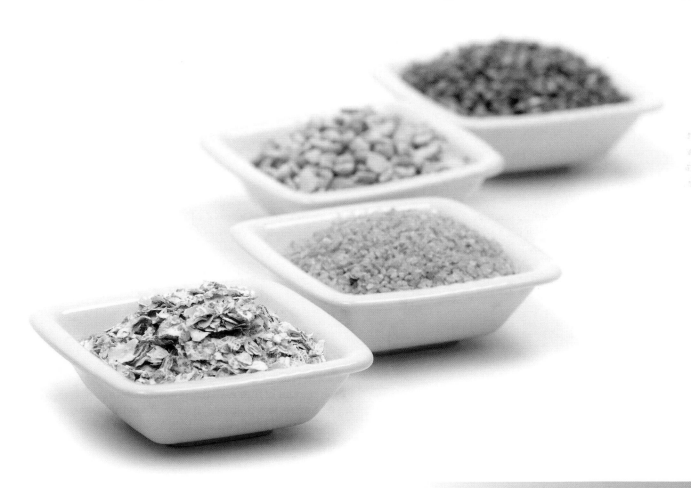

Fruit
–Get Your Daily Dose

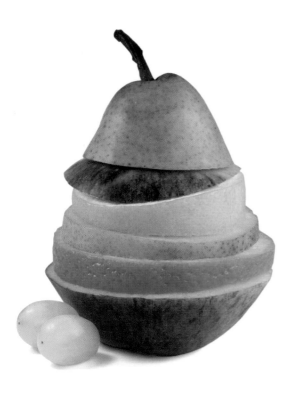

■ Some people claim that you can get fat from fruit. They promise that even a moderate consumption will cause weight gain. However, most people with some knowledge of nutrition know that this is not the case. Fruit contains carbohydrates (10-20 percent), water, fibers, vitamins, antioxidants, minerals, and much more. The only thing that contributes to energy is the carbs, and in light of the fact that most fruits contain only about 10 percent, you would need to eat 2.2 lb (1 kg) of apples to get 3 ½ oz (100 g) of carbs. To get the same number of carbs through bread, you would only need about 7 oz (a couple hundred grams), and from pasta about 10 oz (300 g) (cooked). Because the brain alone uses more than that (an average of 4 ½ oz [120-130 g] of carbohydrates per day), eating a large amount of fruit each day is not a problem.

Of course, it is possible to overeat anything, even fruit, but then again, we would be talking about several *pounds* per day, and as such, you might want to think

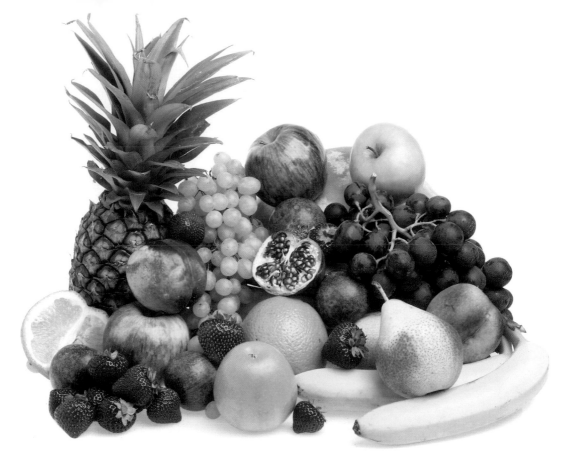

again. Personally, I try to eat about 1 lb (½ kg) of fruit every day, but I'm not afraid to eat double that quantity either. Modern research shows that the more fruit eaten by overweight people, the more they lose weight (193). Even those who are of an average weight can benefit from eating fruit because it also helps protect against weight gain. Research on the subject of fruit intake in relation to body weight shows that fruit has a protective effect against weight gain (198). According to one study, even 100 percent fruit juice does not build fat (192). This is probably due to the high amount of antioxidants, vitamins, and minerals, but also the fibers that help to keep the weight down.

What's So Frightening about Fruit?

Those who are anti-fruit think the scariest thing about fruit is the *fruit sugar* or *fructose*. You can read more about this in the shortcut on carbs on page 17.

Of course, it's true that a large intake of fructose can give you problems because this is a type of sugar that has to be converted in the liver—but you don't have to worry about this when biting into a juicy apple! About half of the sugar in fruit is made up of fructose, so a couple of pounds of fruit a day gives you about 1.75 oz (50 g) of fructose. The liver can take up to 2 ½ oz (75 g) of carbs, and as you rarely eat a couple of pounds of anything at a time, there are never any problems from fructose that comes from fruit. You do not build fat from eating fruit.

However, fructose artificially added to other foods is a different story. If you use fructose as a sweetener, for example, or buy fructose-sweetened candy and drink soda containing a lot of corn syrup high in fructose (this is especially common in the USA), then you easily consume more than the 2 ½ oz (75 g) that the liver can handle. Then the excess gets converted into fat.

Vegetables
–An Effective Fat-Burning Tool

I have worked for many years with clients who want to lose weight. Sometimes they have been participants or cases in some of my lifestyle TV shows and articles I have produced, but often they have been people who come to my nutritional center. The first thing that I do is examine their diet by asking them to keep a thorough food diary. In ninety-nine cases out of a hundred, the intake of fruit and vegetables—especially vegetables—is very small. My standard remedy is to make sure that half of everything they eat during their weight-loss program should consist of vegetables. This means that half their plate will be filled with all sorts of vegetables. They can be raw, cooked, grilled, steamed, prepared in a wok, marinated, or even fried. Of course, this would include the addition of a little bit of oil, but it would still mean a leaner source of protein, a filling meal, and a reasonable caloric intake. Even vegetable juice is good for your weight becuase it fills you up and is low in calories (199).

There isn't much more to add beyond this—this is an easy, nutritional, and very tasty shortcut.

Research Results

> In a Brazilian study, eighty overweight people ate more fruit and vegetables for six months. For every 3 ½ oz (100 g) of vegetables included in the diet, they lost 1.1 lb (0.5 kg) and for every 3 ½ oz (100 g) fruit, 0.6 lb (0.3 kg). With 2 lb (1 kg) more fruit and vegetables per day (half fruit, half vegetables), it should mean a loss of around 17 ½ lb (8 kg) over the course of a year. Just think—it means eating *more* of something, rather than *less*... (194).

> A Spanish study of 206 people showed that weight gain over a ten-year period was less significant for those who mainly ate fruit and vegetables (195). Other studies show similar results (196, 197).

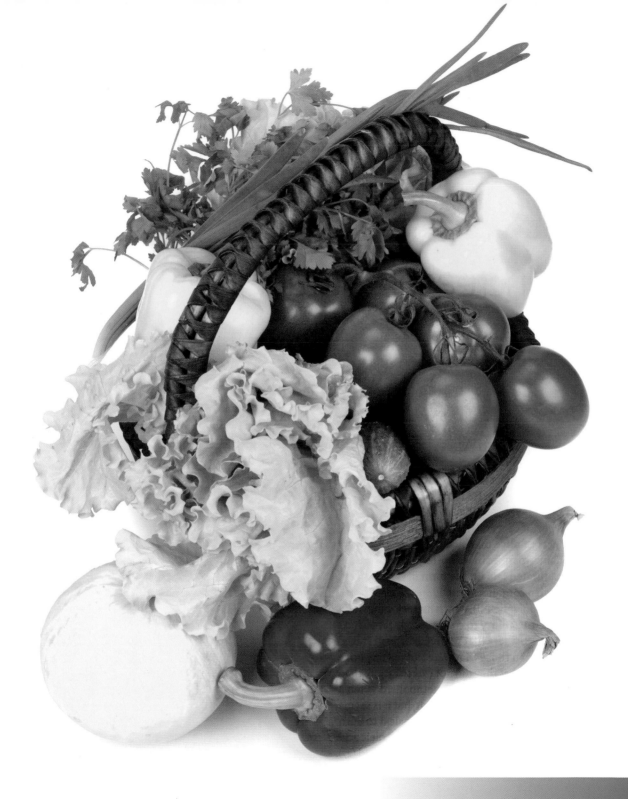

Olive Oil
–For Increased Metabolism

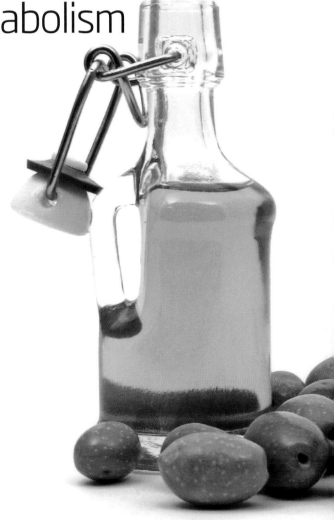

■ Olive oil is probably best known for its role in the Mediterranean diet, famed for its heart healthy properties, a reduced risk of type 2 diabetes, and a lowered risk of certain types of cancer. Newer research has shown that the effects of olive oil reach even into the realm of metabolism. Apart from exceptionally high levels of monounsaturated fats (in the form of 70-80 percent oleic acid), it also contains antioxidants. One of these is oleuropein (a polyphenol), which has been shown in rats to increase the ability to convert body fat to heat (24). This means that rats that received olive oil stayed in better shape than those that were not fed any olive oil, despite the fact that they did not exercise more than the other rats. What happens to metabolism when a human consumes oleuropein is unclear, but it is seems that the fat in olive oil is one of the fats easiest to burn. During exercise, for example, you can see that oleic acid leaves the fat cells more easily and gets metabolized (27).

Olive Oil vs. Sunflower Oil and Linseed Oil

In one study, researchers compared metabolism after eating among groups that consumed either olive oil, sunflower oil, or linseed oil. Olive oil was the type of oil that increased metabolism the most, followed by sunflower oil, and then linseed oil. In these three products, the main fatty acids are oleic acid in olive oil (monounsaturated omega-9 fat), linoleic acid in sunflower oil (polyunsaturated omega-6 fat), and alfa linolenic acid in linseed oil (polyunsaturated omega-3 fat) (25).

Olive Oil vs. Cream

An Australian study looked at the effects on fat burning after a breakfast with 43 percent of calories from fat, with the main fat coming from olive oil or cream. Fat burning was measured five hours following the meal and was shown to be significantly higher for those who were given olive oil. Metabolism was also higher, but only for those people with the most excess weight. Note that dairy fat like cream is not the worst for you when it comes to weight. Dairy fats have about 25 percent SCT and MCT—the types of saturated fats that are easiest to burn. In addition, dairy fats have a decent amount of monounsaturated fats as well as CLA. The difference would probably have been even bigger, and in olive oil's favor, if they had compared it with fat from pork or beef (26).

My View on Olive Oil

In my house, olive oil is the most common source of fat, and there is always an unopened bottle for backup in case the other one runs out. A day sans olive oil isn't easy in my household! We use it with most foods that don't require extremely high temperatures. Obviously, I use it in dressings and to fry at low temperatures. When I use olive oil to coat the pan for frying (when making an omelet, for example), I make sure it doesn't crust or brown, as this damages the nutrients. Olive oil is perfect for baking, and it adds great flavor to stews and other dishes. When preparing leftovers, I'll warm up some rice, grilled chicken breast, and vegetables, flavor it by pouring on some olive oil and bombarding the mix with some of my favorite herbs and spices. Most of these you can read about in the chapter on spices.

When choosing which olive oil to buy at the store, I always go for the one with most color because this means it has the highest level of antioxidants (including the fat-burning inducing oleuropein). Also, I prefer organic olive oil; it tends to have more antioxidants and is not that much more expensive than the conventional one!

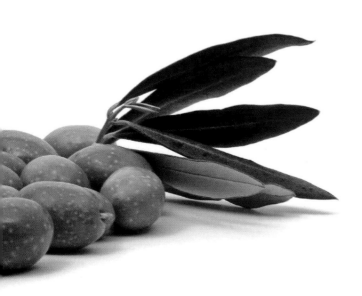

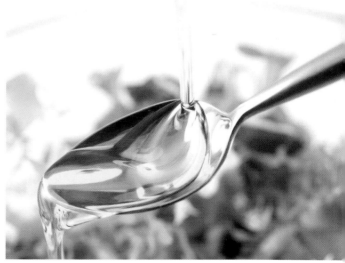

Cocoa

–Not Just Antioxidants...

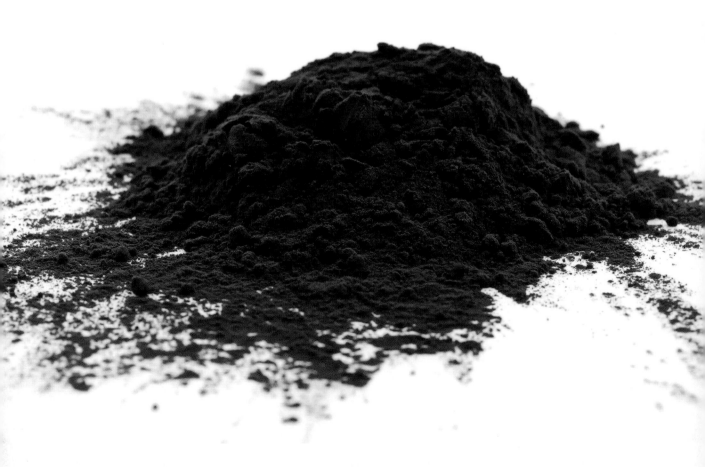

■ Cocoa is known for having extremely high levels of anti-oxidants, mainly in the form of polyphenol. The ORAC score (the unit used to measure antioxidants in food: the higher the better) for cocoa is just over 80,000. Compare this to other healthy foods such as broccoli, which has 1,360, or cashew nuts, with 1,948. Antioxidants are known to maintain the proper level of insulin sensitivity and, therefore, maintain your metabolism.

Cocoa also contains theobromine—a substance that is similar to caffeine, but has a milder effect on the central nervous system. Theobromine is what's poisonous to cats and dogs; they lack the enzymes that are required to break it down. Luckily, humans have enough of those enzymes that the levels of theobromine are not poisonous to us. Moderate amounts of theobromine have also been shown to increase metabolism and the releasing of fat from the fat cells, facilitating a higher fat burning.

Choose the Right Candy

Could we be so lucky that a daily dose of chocolate is a good strategy to increase fat burning and reduce body fat? Unfortunately, this is not the case—at least, not if you choose normal chocolate (milk or dark). In milk and dark chocolate, the calorie content is much larger than the number of calories that the cocoa is able to burn. Cocoa powder and cocoa nibs are much better in this respect because they don't have any added fat or sugar. But, even these give more energy than they use up.

This means that when it comes to burning fat, cocoa should be seen as a better flavor enhancer than other ingredients. But, it's not an active ingredient to help get a firmer body. Most of us want to indulge a little bit now and again, and in terms of body and health, a little piece of dark chocolate is the best option. So, swapping a bowl of chips or a bag of candy for a few squares of dark chocolate can be a useful shortcut. One benefit of dark chocolate is that it's bitter; the bitterness competes with the sweet taste, and this often gets you to stop eating before you get too much excess energy. So, in this way, chocolate is a smarter candy choice, but it's really not one that will make you any fitter.

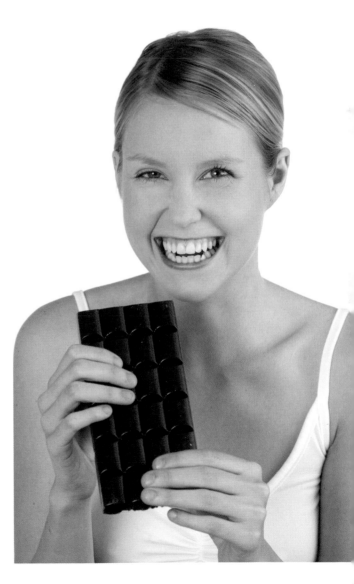

Eggs
–Keep You Full

Eggs are a food often included in breakfast in some manner, whether they are cooked, fried, scrambled, or in an omelet. And, they are a great ingredient if you want to stay full. One study compared how full people felt after a breakfast with either lots of egg or lots of bread. The egg eaters felt fuller and were able to last much better until lunchtime, and they even ate fewer calories during lunch (142)! In addition, they had a more balanced blood sugar level, less insulin, and lower levels of ghrelin. This latter is a hormone that increases appetite and causes cravings for sweet things, so obviously this effect is quite desirable. In another study, a similar result was shown, and here the feeling of fullness was greater—lasting up to thirty-six hours after the breakfast containing eggs (144). This isn't just excellent news for your weight, but is great for your quality of life in general because unhealthy cravings are curbed. In addition, you feel and eat better when you're not starving by lunchtime.

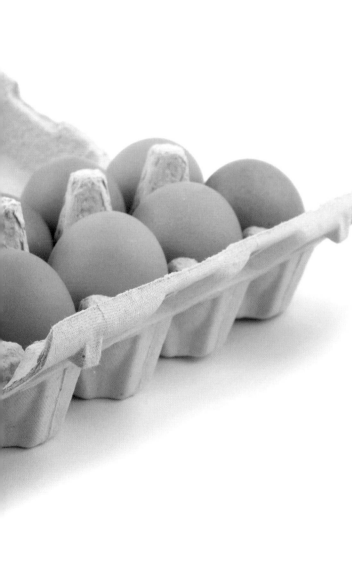

Eggs for Health!

Apart from being filling, eggs are extremely rich in vitamins and minerals, and they can be viewed as a natural daily supplement of vitamin D, zinc, and vitamin B. If you choose omega-3 eggs, you also get those valuable omega-3 fatty acids that have such a stimulating effect on fat burning. Research shows that through eating these eggs instead of normal ones, you can improve your blood lipids and lower your blood sugar (297).

Even the fear of normal eggs and their supposed negative effect on the heart has been reduced in the world of research. Egg yolks do contain some cholesterol (0.2 g) but when you eat them, you lower your own production of cholesterol by the same amount; therefore, the levels of cholesterol are not significant, even when you consume a large quantity of eggs. These days, people are not as concerned by cholesterol's effects on the risk of heart disease. Strictly speaking, you can say that a regular intake of eggs does not increase your risk of heart disease.

My advice? Add an egg or two to your breakfast, eat them as a snack, or make a quick dinner with an omelet.

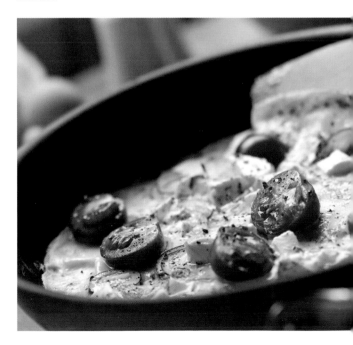

Whole Grain

–Real Food

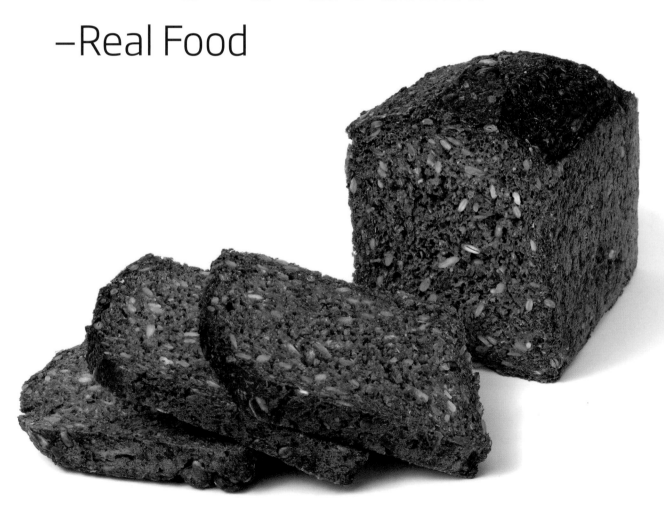

Whole Grain

- Within the range of whole grain products, we can count wholegrain bread, whole wheat pasta, whole grain cereals, and brown rice, as well as flax seeds, quinoa, oatmeal, barley, and rye. The common denominator for all these products is that the seed/grain retains its shell—known as bran—and contains fiber, vitamin B, and trace elements. They even keep the germ, which is packed with vitamins and antioxidants.

  Refined products only keep what is called the endosperm, which only contains carbohydrates, protein, and some fat and only traces of fiber, vitamins, minerals, and antioxidants. To get really nutritious food, you should choose the whole grain alternatives over the refined one. Though there is one drawback to too much whole grain: Sensitive stomachs might protest, so you'll have to find a balance and not overdo your intake of whole grains. As long as your stomach is happy, eating whole grains is good for both your health and your weight.

Whole Grain Encourages Weight Loss

As the whole grain alternatives contain an average of 5-8 percent fewer calories than their refined counterparts, a portion of equal size will be build less fat. Five percent fewer calories might not seem like a lot, but if you consume 2,500 kcal/day and 40 percent of these come from carbohydrates in the form of grains and seeds, it will be around 50 kcal fewer per day (as long as you manage to consume as many of the whole grain varieties as you can). As you might remember from the start of the book, 90 percent of those who gain weight would avoid it completely by consuming 50 kcal fewer per day (162)! We know that those who consume wholegrain products weigh less than others (164, 165, 166, 167, 168), but the real question is whether there are more factors than just a lower calorie content in whole grain.

Why Does Whole Grain Make Us Thin?

It is a known fact that whole grain products are more filling than the same number of calories from refined products. At the same time, it's quite possible that the nutrients in whole grain products also positively affect metabolism; after all, these sorts of products mostly have unsaturated fats, and many antioxidants do positively affect metabolism as well. Even substances with a hormonal effect and a stimulating effect on the metabolism can be found in whole grain products. They also have a higher fiber level, and especially the water-soluble fibers are known to delay a rise in blood sugar after a meal. This gives the food a lower GI value and will be more filling and will make your metabolism more effective.

You can say that whole grain products improve sensitivity to insulin; this is confirmed by the fact that consuming these products gives a measurable reduction in belly fat (305). A low sensitivity to insulin, which is a precursor to type 2 diabetes, is indicated by an apple shaped body—when you gain fat around your stomach. Another property of whole grain is that it increases the release of fat via feces. Between 2 and 10 percent of the fat in food is not absorbed in a meal rich in whole grains (306, 307, 308, 309); this increases the effect of whole grain being more economical with the calories.

Whole Grain Increases Metabolism

Whole grain and food prepared from scratch with high-quality ingredients will have fewer calories and make it easier to feel full. But even more spectacular is the fact that this sort of food increases your metabolism better than refined food. An exciting study compared the increase in metabolism after a snack consisting of either white bread with processed cheese (such as margarine cheese or cream cheese) or whole grain bread with regular cheese. The energy intake was the same, as well as the proportion of fat, protein, and carbs. After this, researchers measured the subjects' metabolism over the course of six hours, and they reached the conclusion that the whole grain bread and the real cheese caused a considerably higher metabolism. The truth is that the whole grain bread increased metabolism twice as much as the white bread (320). A total of 19.9 percent of the whole grain bread's energy content went to digesting the food whereas the white bread only required 10.7 percent of the meal's energy content. If you eat whole grain bread instead of white bread every day, you will see a difference in your waistline, guaranteed.

Grapefruit
–The Appetite Suppressant

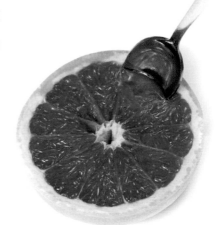

You have probably heard of the grapefruit diet, and it might sound strange, but there is a reason why it's based around just this fruit (even though I strongly advise against diets based on only one type of food).

Grapefruit is a strange food that gives more than just energy, vitamins, minerals, and antioxidants. For a long time, it has been known that the naringin and bergamottin in grapefruits can inhibit the breakdown of certain medicines. The reason for this is that these substances reduce the effect of the enzyme CYP34A, which is important for breaking down many medicines such as Viagra, statins, and immunosuppressants. The effect is so powerful that there is a risk of overdosing on certain substances, and there are documented cases of medicine poisoning from eating just one grapefruit a day. If you take medicine, you should eat grapefruit with some caution and consult your doctor so that you won't be affected by any chemical interactions.

In this case, we are interested in another effect. Grapefruit have been shown to increase metabolism in many ways, and this is, of course, very interesting if you can eat it.

How Does Grapefruit Work?

There seem to be several mechanisms that cause grapefruit to increase metabolism. One possibility is that grapefruit can increase the releasing of fat from the fat cells, but in this case, your body really needs to be in motion to utilize the potential metabolic increase. It's also possible that it can increase metabolism itself, which is likely if you think about the relatively large effect it can have on weight. You can read more about this under the research results heading. A third possibility is that grapefruit suppresses appetite because bitter and sour flavors have a tendency to make you stop eating sooner.

Research Results

> Extract of grapefruit has been shown to increase the releasing of fat from the fat cells. In one study, the subjects consumed a mixture of extracts from blood oranges, oranges, and grapefruit over a period of 12 weeks. They lost 11 ½ oz (5.2 kg) more than the control group (68).

> Another study examined ninety-one overweight people and looked at how either grapefruit concentrate, 8.11 fl oz (240 ml) of grapefruit juice, or half a fresh grapefruit affected sensitivity to insulin and weight. Those who ate the fresh grapefruit lost 3 ½ lb (1.6 kg) after twelve months, whereas those who only drank juice lost 3.3 lb (1.5 kg), and those who got the capsules lost 2.4 lb (1.1 kg). In addition, the sensitivity to insulin increased for those who ate the grapefruit halves, so it's an ideal fruit for people with type 2 diabetes (69).

> Maybe just the taste of grapefruit can contribute to weight loss. A few studies of rats have shown that metabolism increases and appetite is suppressed when rats are exposed to grapefruit oil (70) and/or lemon oil (71). It seems to be a purely neurological effect, which makes the concept of aromatherapy more believable.

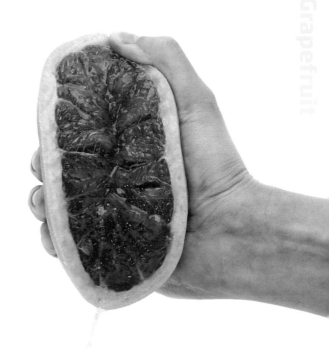

Best Way to Grapefruit!

The best way seems to be to eat half a grapefruit a day. Personally, I prefer a blood orange because it tastes sweeter and contains more antioxidants. Even a daily glass of grapefruit juice is a tasty strategy, but watch out for the more sugary varieties. In Sweden, products called *juice* are supposed to be sugar-free, guaranteed. However, there are also grapefruit drinks that look like juice, but are really just *fruit drinks*.

It's interesting to note that roughly one in ten people have a genetic variation that allows them to taste a flavor in grapefruit that most people cannot. And it tastes horrible to them! So, these people simply can't eat grapefruit or drink grapefruit juice. In this case—and in this case only—a supplement with a grapefruit extract might be a good option to consider.

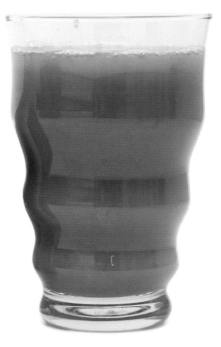

Nuts
–Can Make You Thin

When I was studying to become a nutritionist in the early '90s, nuts were something people were skeptical about. As the most energy laden thing a person could eat, shouldn't they make you fat? A certain amount of vitamins and minerals made them slightly more tolerable, but general advice was to avoid them. So, it was surprising when studies showed that nut lovers actually weigh less than others (145, 147, 148, 155, 156). It soon became clear just how this happens, and although we are still not completely sure how much of a part each factor plays, there are several reasons why nuts help keep your weight stable.

The World's Best Snack

The basal metabolism, or your basic expenditure, is increased by nuts. This is most likely due to the quality of the fat: All nuts contain omega-9 in the form of oleic acid—the same as the main oleic acid found in olive oil. Walnuts also contain omega-3, which we know can raise the basal energy expenditure. Around 10 percent of the energy contained in nuts is thought to be lost through increased energy expenditure (153).

Nuts are very filling per calorie (153), meaning that most people are happy with a few handfuls (1 ¾–3 ½ oz [50–100 g])—a reasonably sized snack that makes it possible to abstain from candy, chocolate bars, and other fat-building snacks. The GI value of nuts is extremely low, so they are one of the best products for balancing blood sugar levels. Interestingly, even adding nuts to dough, for example, lowers the GI value of bread.

Nuts increase sensitivity to insulin, making it easier for the body to burn fat. It's not completely clear what part of the nut causes this effect, but it's likely got something to do with the monounsaturated fats, omega-3, fibers, l-arginine (an amino acid that seems to widen the blood vessels, among other things), and antioxidants (146).

Lower Absorption

You don't absorb all the calories from nuts. Because nuts are hard to chew and difficult to break down completely, some of the fat bypasses the gut. It's thought that around 5-15 percent of the nut's calorie content is lost due to the limited absorption (153). Research also shows that the number of times you chew has a considerable effect on absorption. One study showed that chewing forty times had a greater effect on absorption than chewing only twenty-five times, which in turn was more effective than ten times (151).This should not be seen as a reason to chew sloppily because doing so can

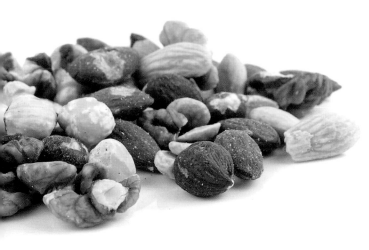

cause stomach problems and a lower rate of nutrient absorption. But, nevertheless, it's interesting that nuts are so heavily affected by chewing.

Research Results

> In a study of fifty insulin-resistant people, half included 1 oz (30 g) of natural nuts per day in their diet over the span of twelve weeks. The nut portion consisted of ½ oz (15 g) walnuts, ¼ oz (7.5 g) almonds, and ¼ oz (7.5 g) hazelnuts. Despite the small quantity, the group that ate the nuts showed an improvement in insulin sensitivity and, therefore, a decrease in insulin secretion (149).

> A huge study of 51,188 nurses aged 20–45 years showed that two or more portions of nuts per week better reduced the risk of weight gain when compared with those who ate nuts less frequently. The study lasted eight years, and this protective effect applied to both those who were of an average weight and those who were overweight (150). Similar effects have also been noted in other studies (154).

> In one study, twenty women ate the equivalent of 350 kcal per day of almonds over a period of ten weeks. They received all the heart healthy benefits of the almonds, but did not gain weight. A number of subjects pointed to the fact that the almonds were so filling that they had no problem refraining from eating the same amount of energy from unhealthier foods (157).

> In another study of the effects of almonds on twenty-seven men with high cholesterol, researchers wanted to check the effect of nuts on insulin secretion. Subjects were divided into three groups and received either 1.3 oz (36 g) or 2.6 oz (73 g) of almonds a day over the course of a month. The third group was the control group in which the men received no almonds at all. Both the groups that ate almonds had lower levels of insulin secretion during a period of twenty-four hours, showing that as little as an ounce (30 g) of almonds a day is enough to achieve this effect. Because insulin has a negative effect on blood fats, increases the risk for type 2 diabetes, and makes us fat, this is good information to know (158).

> In another study, researchers examined the effect on weight and health when consuming either 3 oz (84 g) of almonds a day or the equivalent amount of slow-release carbohydrates. Sixty-five overweight subjects, divided into two groups, kept a low calorie diet over the course of twenty-four weeks; both groups ate the same number of calories. We know that slow-release carbs are beneficial to weight, but the almonds actually had a better effect. Those who ate almonds saw their BMI sink by 18 percent, as opposed to the 11 percent for those eating slow-release carbs. The amount of fat was reduced by 30 percent as opposed to 20 percent, and the waistline was reduced on average by 14 percent, compared to 9 percent for those who didn't eat almonds. In addition, almonds seemed to lower blood pressure by 11 percent, whereas the other group did not see their blood pressure affected (159).

> Does eating too many walnuts affect weight gain? To answer that question, ninety subjects ate a quantity of walnuts equivalent to 130 kcal above their daily energy requirement every day for a period of six months. In theory, this should lead to a 7.5 lb (3.4 kg) weight increase, but in practice, there was hardly any weight gain at all. The BMI increased by a negligible 0.1 units (160).

Peanuts
–Nutritionally Better Than You Think

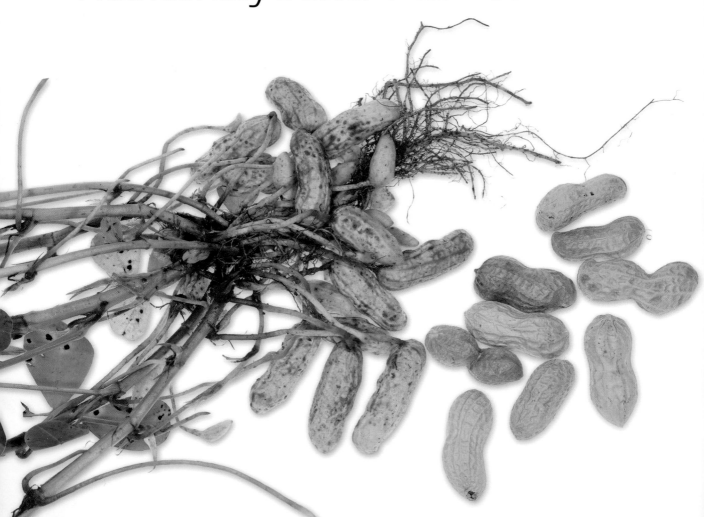

At seminars and exhibitions, I am often asked if peanuts are as good as other nuts, and it's always asked in such a way as if the answer is expected to be "no." Many people associate peanuts with beer, soda, Snickers bars, chips, and other unhealthy foods, so they're always surprised when I explain that peanuts are great for keeping in shape when eaten in moderation. This is because peanuts are rich in protein—they're almost 30 percent protein. In addition, the fat in peanuts consists mainly of monounsaturated fats—the same as in other nuts, olive oil, and avocado—and is relatively easy for the body to burn off. Peanuts even have some lineolic acid, which has one of the most stimulating effects on metabolism that we know of. Also, peanuts (just like red wine) contain resveratrol which has been shown, at least in animal studies, to increase metabolism (203). But, it's unclear how effective the dosage found in peanuts is. Peanuts have very few carbs and those that are present have a very low GI value.

Much Better Than Candy

Botanically speaking, peanuts are legumes, but as the nutrient content and structure is so similar to nuts, it's not surprising that they can help us maintain our weight (152). A Swedish study tested to see what happened when twenty-five people ate either too much candy or too many peanuts. The excess amount of energy was the same, (20 kcal/kg body weight) but only the candy group saw their waistline increase. One explanation was that the basal energy expenditure only increased for the peanut group (around a 5-percent increase), so even if the peanuts are roasted and salted, they are still the better snacking alternative and are significantly better than chips or cheese puffs.

How Should Peanuts be Consumed?

We have raw peanuts, roasted and salted, or roasted and unsalted peanuts, honey-roasted peanuts, and peanut butter, and the question is if there is a difference in their effect on our body weight. To investigate this, researchers asked 118 subjects to eat 2 oz (56 g) of one of these peanut products each day for four weeks (204). In the end, not even those who ate the honey-roasted peanuts gained any weight (no significant weight gain was seen in any group) and LDL (known as bad cholesterol) was lowered for all subjects. In addition, HDL (good cholesterol) was raised, and the triglycerids were lowered; this makes me want to credit peanuts of all varieties (except puffed and processed peanuts) with protecting against heart disease. I also want to put them on par with other nuts when it comes to their effect on weight because they do have many similar properties.

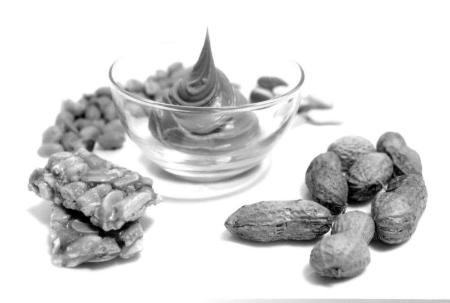

Super Soy
–Great for Your Shape

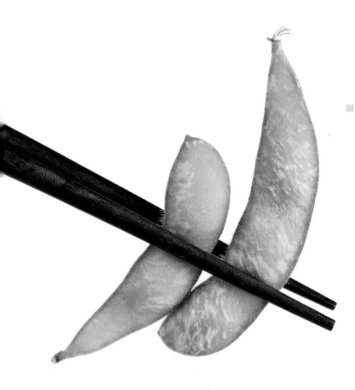

Legumes such as beans, lentils, and peas are great for keeping in shape due to their low GI, high levels of protein, and large proportion of fibers. However, the legume that has received the most attention when it comes to burning fat is the soybean. It's readily available and can be used in many ways. The soybean has a distribution of nutrients that is very similar to that recommended by the iso diet, and it's suitable for use as a basic ingredient in salads, stews, etc. The soybean's protein level is among the highest of all legumes, and the combination of fatty acids, with a high proportion of unsaturated fats, is very good for burning fat. Research also shows that exchanging some of your caloric intake from one type of food for the same amount of calories from soy usually leads to weight loss (210). The reason for this is not clear, but it must either mean that you don't absorb the calories from soy as effectively, or that soy increases your metabolism.

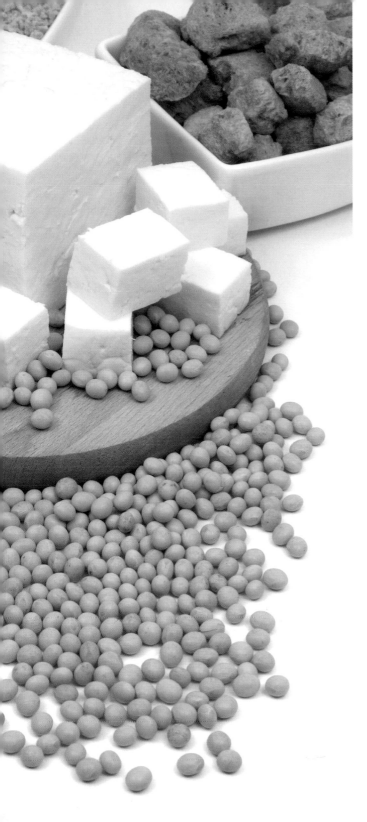

Soybeans When Dieting

One of the big problems with dieting is that the body lowers its metabolism when you decrease your energy intake. It's a survival mechanism that works by reducing the amount of thyroid hormone (T3) when you eat less. T3 steers your metabolism, so when this is lowered, you also reduce your energy levels and the amount of calories your body needs each day.

A lot of research points to the fact that if you eat soy while dieting, you can help keep T3 levels up despite a reduced energy intake (207). The result should be an increase in both weight loss and energy.

Research also shows that the isoflavonoids in soy enable you to burn fat more effectively while keeping your muscle mass at the same time. The isoflavonoids are the same as phytoestrogen, but don't be fooled by the term "estrogen." Even though it's chemically reminiscent of estrogen, it does not always have the same effect as the female hormone. One study showed that the consumption of soy proteins with extra isoflavonoids produces less body fat and more muscle, compared to milk proteins that produce the same amount of protein, but lack the isoflavonoids found in soy (208).

Soy products have various properties that make them suitable for a diet, and it seems as though when eaten regularly, they can counteract weight gain. In one Hawaiian study, researchers looked at the consumption of soy by 1,418 women over a period of time; those who ate the most soy tended to have the lowest BMI (209). Another very positive effect of soy is that it protects your bone density when you diet (210). Losing bone density increases the risk of osteoporosis, which is not uncommon when dieting.

The best soy products are soybeans, soy protein powders, soy mince, soy sausages, soy meatballs, etc. It's important that the amount of soy protein be adequate. Please note that soy sauce only contains trace amounts of soybeans and does not count as an effective source.

The Iso Diet
–Your Optimal Fat-Burning Method

■ I have worked with health and nutrition since the late '80s, and I've read most studies of any value on the subjects of weight loss and metabolism. In addition, I have worked with clients who come to my nutrition center, and I have helped numerous people get in shape since the late 1980s. With my colleagues Martin Brunnberg and Kristina Andersson, I have selected the best and most-documented factors that affect us; we call it the *iso diet*. The name comes from the Greek "iso," meaning equal parts, and "dietos," meaning daily diet. In the iso diet, you eat equal parts of calories from fat, protein, and carbohydrates every day, and this proportionate way of eating makes it easy to either maintain your weight or lose weight because the food is both filling and increases your metabolism. If you exercise as well as follow the iso diet, the fat will be used as fuel instead of filling up the fat cells.

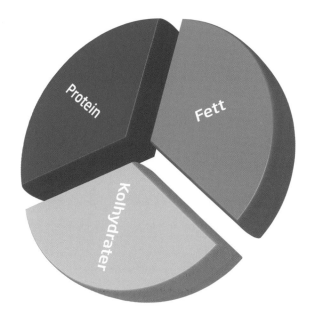

What Does the Iso Diet Consist of?

The iso diet's main ambition is that you should feel full on the right amount of calories in order to lose weight. This means that the programs that can be found in books and on the official iso diet website recommend about 1600 kcal/day, which is less than most people expend.

A normal amount of energy expenditure for an average active woman is 2,200 kcal; for a man with a similar level of activity, it is 2,800 kcal. With the iso diet, this means you eat less than you use up (this is the basis of all diets), but as you are eating foods that have been documented to have the most filling effect, you won't be fighting your hunger all day.

In addition, with the iso diet, you can eat up to five meals per day. Breakfast, lunch, dinner, and two snacks—and this means that you never get the chance to feel especially hungry between meals. That intense craving that comes from the "reptilian brain" never comes. And, as we know, the reptilian brain is activated when we're hungry, and it's very hard to withstand. It craves fat and sugar, and this is what you end up feeding it. The different meals in the iso diet are perfectly balanced and take into account both energy content as well as the combination of nutrients.

One-Third Protein

According to the iso diet, you should eat 33 percent of calories from protein; this is a lot more than the average person eats—often around 15 percent of calories from protein.

You can read about what happens when you increase your protein intake on page 18, but in essence it goes like this: You feel full on fewer calories, while at the same time you increase your metabolism. In addition, the body becomes keen to burn fat, so if you exercise regularly, you can fully utilize this increased potential (189).

Thanks to the iso diet's high protein intake, you will not lose muscle (a side effect of other diets in which both fat and muscle are reduced). Keeping your muscle is also good for your metabolism and health, and it looks great!

One-Third Fat

We have long known that we burn more fat when we increase our consumption of fat. When the body knows that there is a good source of fat, it does not feel the need to store any, and instead works towards burning it off. Fat is also filling and delays the emptying of the stomach, meaning that your blood sugar is stable, and you can easily last until your next meal.

Therefore, the key to keeping a low body fat is to include some fat in your diet. But, you have to make sure that it's the right fat and the right amount because it is the most energy-loaded nutrient with its 9 kcal/gram. For example, if you burn 2,000 kcal/day but increase your fat consumption so that your intake is 2,500 kcal/day, it won't matter how high your metabolism is. You'll still have 500 kcal extra each day, and this excess will lead to weight gain. If about a third of the food's calories are from fat, there won't be an excess of energy, just enough to keep the fat-burning process going.

The Right Fats: A Quick Run-Through

In shortcuts 3-5, you read about the different fats and their various fat-burning and fat-storing properties. The only fats that are completely banned in the iso diet are synthetic trans fats. CLA is also a trans fat, but it's natural and is mostly beneficial. Synthetic trans fats lower your sensitivity to insulin and are more likely to be stored as fat. They are present in foods that you already know are bad for you: Some cookies, candy, some margarines, baked goods, ice cream, snacks, frozen foods, sauce mixes, and oils for deep-fat frying. They are often described as "partially hydrogenated," and they're easy to avoid if you keep your eyes open for them. Cooking from scratch, as recommended by the iso diet, enables you to stay away from these without any problems. The fats we focus on are omega-3 (EPA, DHA, and DPA), omega-9 (oleic acid), and the short- and medium-chained saturated fats (SCT and MCT). Long-chained saturated fats (LCT) appear in smaller amounts in the iso diet, mainly due to the fact that they contain fat-storing properties. That they exist naturally in most products is fine because they appear in such small amounts.

One-Third Carbohydrates

Simple math shows us that the last third of energy intake comes from carbohydrates. This enables you to keep your brain going and have enough energy to exercise. In addition, it's important for your immune system. Food with carbs gives you a number of other nutrients such as vitamins, minerals, fibers, and antioxidants.

The iso diet is a type of low-carb diet because it doesn't give you enough carbs to inhibit fat burning or have a negative effect on your health. Compare this to an average person, who gets roughly half his or her energy intake from carbs. Because the iso diet also decreases your energy intake, the amount of carbs consumed is even less than if you ate 33 percent of calories from carbs as part of a normal energy intake. And, of course, all carbs in this program have a low GI, meaning that they are absorbed slowly by the body and provide a maximum feeling of fullness, with minimal secretion of insulin. As we already know, this keeps the fat burning.

What Do the Meals Look Like?

With all the knowledge we have about how our body clock affects the way nutrients are handled by the body, the meals all look slightly different. The point is that you consume more carbs and energy early on in the day and less of these the later it becomes. A typical day can look like the one listed below, but please note that you should adapt the timing to your personal needs.

Breakfast: Fruit with Egg and Cheese
390 kcal, 37 E% (percent of energy) fat, 31 E% carbohydrates, 32 E% protein

2 eggs
1.75 oz (50 g) firm cheese, 10% fat
8.8 oz (250 g) berries or fruit

Boil the eggs and slice the cheese into batons. Eat together with the fruit.

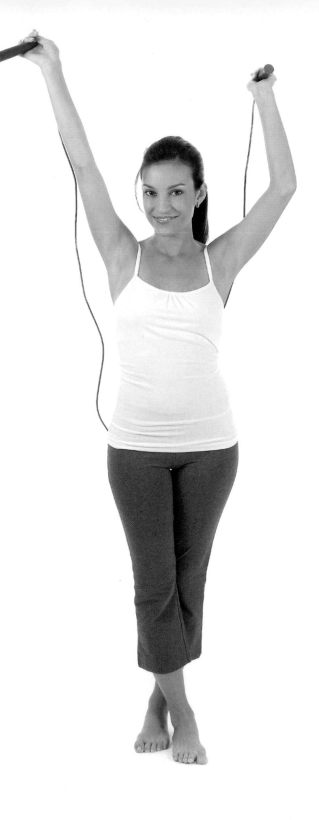

Snack 1: Apple with Cottage Cheese, Almonds, and Cinnamon

155 kcal, 38 E% fat, 28 E% carbohydrates, 34 E% protein

> 3 ½ oz (100 g) cottage cheese
> 5 (5 g) almonds
> ½ (65 g) apple, finely chopped
> Cinnamon

Mix the cottage cheese with the finely chopped apple and almonds. Sprinkle some cinnamon on top and enjoy!

Lunch: Cooked Salmon with a Bean and Vegetable Mix

490 kcal, 34 E% fat, 32 E% carbohydrates, 34 E% protein

> 4 oz (120 g) salmon
> 1 can (400 g) crushed or whole tomatoes
> 5 oz (150 g) boiled/canned broad beans
> 2 garlic cloves
> Fresh chili pepper to taste
> A pinch of parsley

Poach the salmon in water for 5–7 minutes until cooked through. Pour tomatoes in a pan and heat while stirring. Add the beans, pressed or chopped garlic, and the chopped chili peppers and parsley. Add salt to taste. Warm through and serve with the salmon. Done in fifteen minutes!

Snack 2: A Snack Salad

155 kcal, 35 E% fat, 28 E% carbohydrates, 37 E% protein

> 1 ¾ oz (50 g) spinach
> 1.4 oz (40 g) salad leaves of your choice
> Half a pepper (30 g)
> 4 (8 g) walnuts
> 1 oz (30 g) firm cheese, 10% fat
> Half a pear (65 g)
> 1 ¾ oz (50 g) pea shoots

Place the spinach and salad evenly on a plate. Cut the pepper into batons, and add to the plate. Crush the nuts, slice the cheese and pear into pieces, and place on top of the other ingredients. Top off with the pea shoots.

Dinner: Chicken Kabobs with Peanuts and Root Vegetables

395 kcal, 37 E% fat, 21 E% carbohydrates, 42 E% protein

> 4.4 oz (125 g) chicken breast (preferably corn-fed chicken)
> 1 small (70 g) celeriac
> 1 small (70 g) beetroot
> ½ (70 g) rutabaga
> ½ (75 g) kohlrabi
> About 30 (30 g) peanuts

Cut the chicken into one inch (2 x 2 cm) pieces, and place on a skewer. Cut the root vegetables into pieces, and place in an ovenproof dish; place the chicken skewers on top. Bake in the oven at 390°F (200°C) for about 25 minutes or until cooked through. Sprinkle with peanuts before serving.

The Iso Diet as a Lifestyle

Personally, I eat according to the same principles recommended by the iso diet, and I love many of the foods included in this diet. However, I don't follow a specific program because I don't need to lose weight. My meals don't follow a specific portion size, but have a similar spread of nutrients. The right fat is a must, and I decrease the amount of carbs I eat in the evening. This is how easy it is to have the iso diet as part of your lifestyle. It's even easy to stick to the iso diet while eating out at a restaurant. Just ask the wait staff to modify the portions so that there is less pasta, rice, or potato and a little more fish, meat, or poultry. Even diabetics can benefit from the iso diet, and we have seen many cases of those with both type 1 and type 2 diabetes who have better controlled their blood sugar levels with this method of eating. Interestingly, the Joslin Diabetes Center (affiliated with Harvard University) recommends a diet with 30 percent of calories from protein, 30 percent of calories from fat, and 40 percent of calories from carbohydrates for those who have type 2 diabetes, and as well as for those looking to prevent diabetes. As you can see, this is very similar to the iso diet (201)!

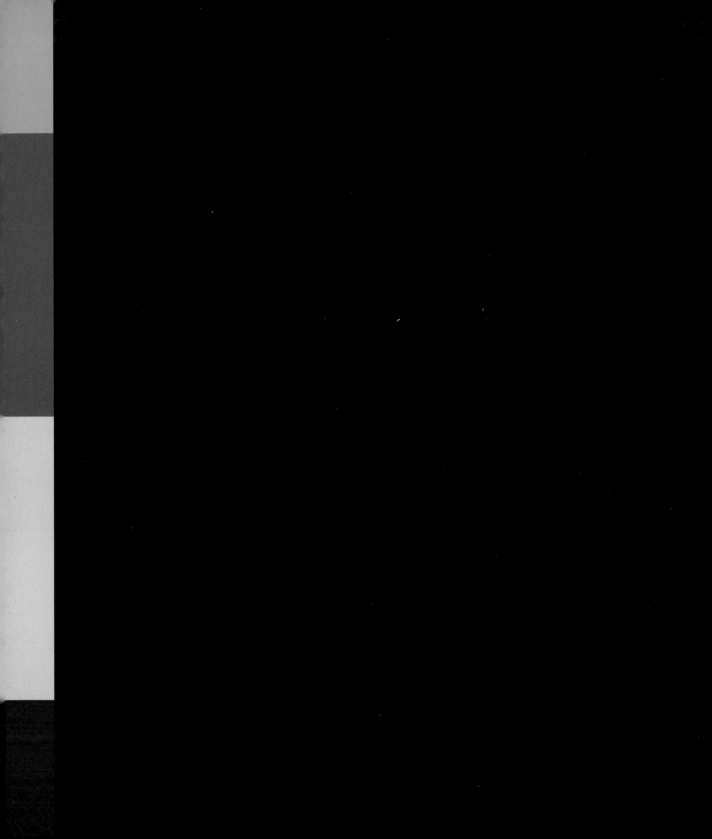

Drink Efficiently and Burn Fat

Tea
–Black, White, and Green

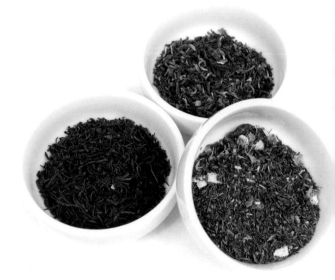

It wasn't that long ago that tea was seen as a stimulant, something of an addiction, and a little bit naughty—certainly not something that could contribute to better health and fitness. But sure enough, scientific reports emerged about tea's excellent qualities. Most studies focused on green tea, but even black, white, and oolong tea appear to have a positive effect on both fat burning and metabolism.

At least two of the ingredients in tea have an effect—the *methylxanthines* (caffeine and theobromine), and a form of antioxidant known as *catechins*, known in tea as EGCG. Research has shown very interesting effects, such as EGCG's ability to increase the liver's metabolism, so that you are "fueling the fire" and losing calories without having to exercise. EGCG also inhibits lipases in your small intestine, leading to reduced fat absorption. Some of the fat you eat will simply disappear down the toilet, and you'll end up with a lower energy intake.

In one study, 1/3 cup (750 ml) of oolong tea caused a loss of nearly .70 oz (20 g) of fat during a trial meal (59). This is equivalent to 180 kcal/day if it's a daily habit; after a year, this adds up to the dizzying amount of 65,700 kcal that end up down the toilet. Unfortunately, the polyphenols don't distinguish between types of fat, so make sure you eat enough omega-3 fatty acids, for example, to cover your needs.

Tea Before Dinner?

Another interesting effect of tea (and warm, calorie-free drinks in general) is that they increase your core temperature (i.e., in the torso and around the liver) when you drink them. By this I mean the temperature in the torso and around the liver; When the temperature rises, it suppresses your appetite. Even caffeine and theobromine can increase body temperature and contribute to this effect; it's similar to what you might experience during the summer when the weather is warm and you have less of an appetite. The liver's metabolism will increase due to the effect of the EGCG, and the heat in the drink will suppress your appetite. This means a cup of green tea before your meal will suppress your appetite, and you will feel full on a smaller amount of food.

Tea and Exercise

One of the positive benefits of tea for those who enjoy exercising is that it gives you an energy boost and makes working out feel a bit easier. Some research shows that tea's fat-burning properties are increased through exercise. One American study showed that both the subcutaneous fat in the stomach and the fat that can be found in the abdominal cavity (your paunch) were easier to burn off for those who were already fit and had an intake of EGCG and caffeine (3). This is not surprising because caffeine releases fat from the fat cells, so that it can be metabolized rather than stored.

Caffeine, Theobromine, and Theanine

Just under a cup (200 ml) of tea contains ¾-1 ¾ oz (20-50 g) of caffeine—considerably less than a cup of coffee, which can contain 2.8-5.3 oz (80-150 mg) of caffeine depending on the strength. Not only does caffeine increase the metabolic functions of the liver and keep the body temperature high, it also increases your total energy expenditure without any extra exercise. If, however, you do choose to exercise, the caffeine will stimulate the release of fat from the fat cells, resulting in the fat going to your muscles to be burned. This makes it easier to keep your performance levels high while simultaneously burning fat that would otherwise remain stored. Caffeine is also an energy enhancer, meaning that you can exercise more often using more effort. This increases fat burning and gives your workout better results. Theobromine has an effect similar to caffeine, but it's a slightly weaker stimulant. (You can read more about theobromine in shortcut 14.) Some people feel that they can drink tea late at night without affecting their sleep; this could be due to an amino acid called theanine, which seems to

reduce the restlessness that caffeine causes. This is a plus if you enjoy drinking tea late at night, but it's a drawback when it comes to getting an energy lift.

Research Results

Because of the many studies on tea and body weight, it's hard to give an exact number when it comes to how much body fat you will have after a month of drinking tea. There's also some variation between types of tea, how often you drink it, and the quantity consumed. However, here are a few examples from a handful of studies.

> 102 overweight subjects drank tea made from about four teabags (8 g) of oolong tea leaves every day for six weeks. Seventy percent of the subjects lost more than 2.2 lb (1 kg), and 22 percent lost more than 6 ½ lb (3 kg), so the effect seems to depend on the individual (2).

> 60 overweight subjects from Thailand drank either green tea or a placebo every day during a twelve-week diet, and the difference between the groups was roughly 7.3 lb (3.3 kg) lost by the end of the study. The researchers also measured the metabolism of the two groups, and the tea drinkers used roughly 45 kcal/day more than those who drank the placebo. In addition, a slightly larger proportion of the energy expenditure came from fat with the tea drinkers (4).

Do Supplements with EGCGs Work?

In theory, a supplement with EGCG should give the same effect as an equivalent amount in tea, but in practice, EGCG seems to work best in liquid form. The caffeine in tea seems necessary for the EGCG's beneficial effects, and this was shown in an analysis of fifteen different studies on green tea and body weight (1). EGCG together with caffeine gave both a lower BMI and body weight, whereas on its own, EGCG was less effective. If you want to take EGCG as a supplement, you need to double check that the supplement contains caffeine. But, why not just drink tea instead? It's cheaper, tastier, and the effect is guaranteed. In addition, it contains several still unknown substances that might be proven effective.

Coffee
–A Great-Tasting Metabolism Booster

■ Coffee is one of the world's most consumed drinks, and researchers instinctively seem to think it's unhealthy. This seems logical because it stimulates the central nervous system and is made from roasted beans—all forms of roasting are considered to create substances that can cause damage.

Coffee is also one of the most studied foods, and a search of the word "coffee" in medical databases brings up several thousand hits. But, what's interesting is that very few of these writings are negative. Of course, some people have problems falling asleep if they drink coffee too late, and it is a diuretic, which can irritate sensitive bladders, but no one *has* to drink coffee late at night, and it actually gives you more fluids than you lose. Too much coffee can, of course, give you heart palpitations and the shakes, but just about everything causes side effects when consumed in excess.

On the plus side, if you consume an average amount of coffee, there are a host of benefits, including lowered risk of depression, protection against certain forms of cancer (including skin cancer and intestinal cancer), a reduced risk of cirrhosis of the liver and other liver damage, a reduced risk of heart disease and type 2 diabetes, a heightened cognitive ability amongst the elderly, and, of course, feeling more alert. This last one can literally be a life-saver—for example, if you're driving a car. However, the reason coffee is part of this book is because it also gets your metabolism going.

How Does Coffee Work?

Firstly, you can almost guarantee that those who drink coffee weigh less than those who don't (60). There are many reasons, such as the heat in coffee, which reduces appetite—an effect of warm drinks, such as tea. Caffeine also releases dopamine, a neurotransmitter that works on the reward center in the brain. We need dopamine to feel good. It's also released by other components of food, such as fat, sugar, and alcohol. Because we need to get dopamine from some source, it's possible that drinking coffee satisfies this need and allows you to stick to foods with fewer calories. In essence, you're drinking coffee instead of eating candy or drinking calorie-laden drinks.

But, maybe caffeine contains other properties that boost metabolism.

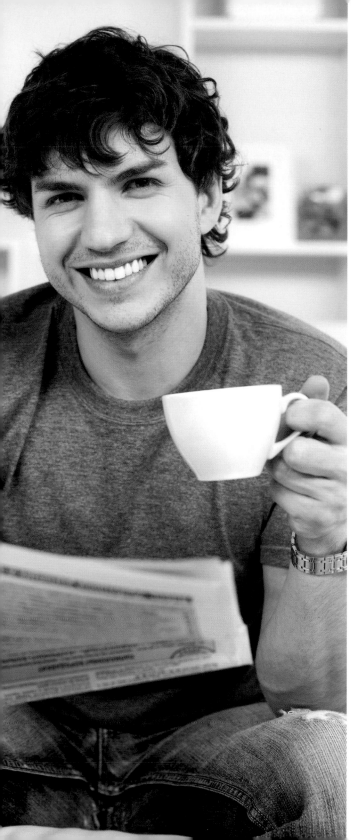

Caffeine: A Double-Edged Sword

If you ingest caffeine in the form of tablets or as an energy drink, it will drastically lower your sensitivity to insulin (61), which is the first step toward type 2 diabetes. Strangely enough, though, coffee seems to have the opposite effect; it's been discovered that coffee has a very strong protective effect against type 2 diabetes (62), and the more coffee you drink, the lower the risk seems to be. A lower risk of type 2 diabetes also means a better metabolism and lower body weight.

Caffeine consumed the right way has two positive effects on metabolism. Firstly, it increases the liver's metabolic effect, thermogenesis, and secondly, it releases fat from the fat cells to enable a better rate of fat burning.

The studies are clear in their message: If you want to burn fat and keep healthy, you should ingest caffeine in the form of tea or coffee—and nothing else. Forget energy drinks and caffeine pills! Worst-case scenario, these can reduce your sensitivity to insulin and, long-term, can have a negative effect on fat burning. Energy drinks especially are notorious for this because in addition to caffeine, they contain massive quantities of sugar.

Chlorogenic Acid: Scary Name, Cool Effect

One of the active substances in coffee is chlorogenic acid. Despite the fact that it sounds like some kind of biological warfare, it's actually very healthy. One of its effects is to delay the absorption of glucose from the small intestine (starch is broken down to glucose in the small intestine) (67). The result is a slower rise in blood sugar and a reduced secretion of insulin.

However, coffee contains a veritable cocktail of chemical substances that can have a variety of effects. One of these substances, which also seems to delay the uptake of glucose in the intestines, is the alkaloid trigonelline. This is chemically related to caffeine, but it has completely different effects (65).

Even many forms of antioxidants are present in coffee, such as phenols, which are proven to be good for health and metabolism.

Research Results

> One study of 1,141 healthy Americans aged 45–74 years showed that the higher the daily consumption of coffee, the lower the BMI. The group that drank 12 (!) or more cups a day had a 67 percent lower risk of getting type 2 diabetes as compared to those who drank no coffee at all (62).

> A large scientific examination of 18 studies that took place between 1966 and 2009 showed that both decaffeinated coffee and normal coffee had a protective effect against type 2 diabetes. This shows that the properties that protect against diabetes are beyond just the caffeine in coffee. A total of 457,922 subjects were studied, so there was a wealth of material. And every cup of coffee consumed reduced the risk of type 2 diabetes by 7 percent. Because type 2 diabetes increases the amount of stored fat, this is an important effect with regard to weight (63).

> A smaller study that looked at the effect of pure caffeine (10 mg/kg body weight) over the course of four hours showed that metabolism increased by 13 percent during the fourth hour. In addition, the release of fat from the fat cells increased by 100 percent, which wouldn't be of interest if these fats then returned to the cells, rather than being burned in the liver or muscles. However, the results showed that 24 percent of the fat was metabolized, which is a definite increase when compared to the amount of fat burning before the caffeine was consumed (64).

Which Coffee Is Best?

Good old filter coffee is best when it comes to health and, of course, it should be drunk without sweetener. If you want some milk, my advice would be to use a dash of skim milk. When you choose to use cream in your coffee, the caloric intake of drinking even one cup of coffee a day with a splash of cream would be enormous over the course of a year, and would be equivalent to many pounds of body weight.

Boil coffee (a coarser grind) tends to impair the blood fats, whereas instant coffee is more refined, and some of the antioxidants are lost. Many instant coffees are also flavored with sugar and various cream substitutes, as well as flavorings; these products are hugely caloric, and they can even contain trans fats. I recommend buying filter coffee that has been mildly roasted because the heating process during roasting damages the antioxidants.

The latest on the coffee front is the so-called *green coffee* in which some of the beans are not roasted. This makes it a healthier drink with a milder taste. Maybe it will become as popular as green tea?

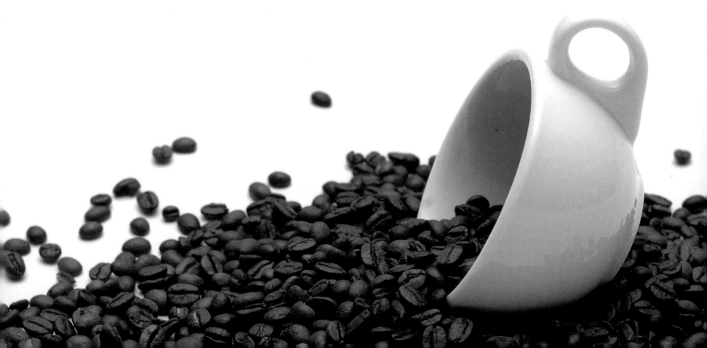

Water
–The Best Mealtime Drink

What is the cheapest drink in the world that's also healthy and perfect with all meals? Water, of course! And as a bonus, there are even several ways in which water can make you thin. Obviously, the first way is by exchanging other drinks, such as juice, soda, beer, or milk, with water at mealtimes. All of these drinks contain energy, and liquid calories are known to be poor at giving you that feeling of being full. The worst are sugary drinks such as soda and juice because they don't fill you up but give you about 400 kcal per quart (liter). If you eliminate your daily consumption of a liter of soda, you'll reduce excess calories by the equivalent of 44 lb (20 kg) of body fat per year! No wonder it's so easy to drink yourself fat.

Also, the fact that water fills your stomach (without contributing a single calorie!) means that you'll eat less when you drink a large glass of water with your meal.

Water Balances Blood Sugar

It used to be believed that you shouldn't drink water with your meal because it will dilute the stomach and pancreatic juices and give you a reduced nutrient absorption. This, however, is wrong. We have enough enzymes to break down an enormous amount of food, so the absorption is just as effective. It will, however, be slower if we drink water with our meal! The reason for this is that the contents of our intestines increase, which means that the blood sugar is slower to rise. As we know, this results in a more stable blood sugar level, which suppresses appetite, reduces dangerous sugar highs, and lowers insulin levels. And because insulin builds fat, this last effect is very important. Therefore, you should drink at least a cup (300 ml) of water with your meal.

Water Increases Metabolism

Because water has no calories, it's interesting that the metabolism of water in the body actually uses up energy. There is no food that can be considered to contain negative calories, whereby food takes more energy to metabolize than its caloric value. But, water comes fairly close because it doesn't add any calories at all.

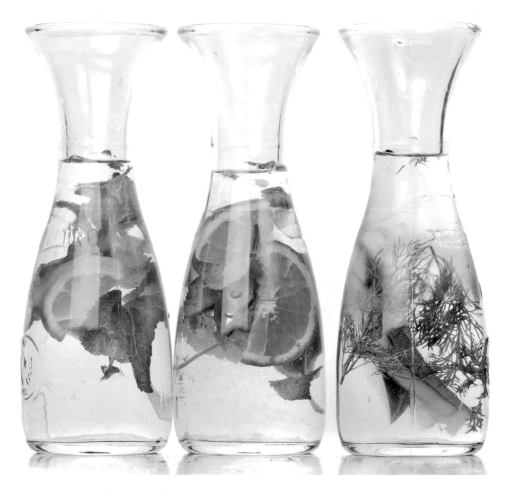

To drink a quart (liter) of water will increase your metabolism by about 10 calories per day. It might not sound like much, but once again, it adds up over a year. You can read exactly how big this effect is later one. However, drinking 5-10 quarts (5-10 liter) of water to increase your metabolism is not a good idea because this can have a negative effect on your health. Consuming too much water in too short a time span is actually fatal because your bodily fluids become diluted, and the balance of minerals gets disrupted. Even a more moderate overconsumption can have negative effects, such as incontinence and diarrhea, so please be sensible. About 2 quarts (2 liters) spread out over the course of the day (depending on the temperature and how active you are) is normally sufficient for most people.

Water Increases Fat Burning

Your body can tell how good your fluids are, and if you're slightly dehydrated, your body will be less likely to release fats from the fat cells (43, 44). An increased level of free fatty acids in the blood when you are dehydrated can be dangerous because the blood will be less viscous, and the risk for thrombosis will increase. Therefore, the release of fats from the fat cells is only effective when you are well hydrated. Because the metabolism in the liver and muscles requires that fatty acids move from the fat cells into the blood before being able to enter the cells that are to metabolize them, a reduced release of fatty acids is the same as a reduced metabolism. Research shows that the release of fat gradually decreases when we are dehydrated and increases when we drink enough. If you do endurance training, it's very important for your performance that you keep well hydrated, so make sure you drink at every opportunity. Dehydration has been shown to increase muscle wastage (43), which is definitely not something you want because muscles are active parts of your body that burn fat, even at rest. If you want to watch your weight, you need to keep your muscles strong. This means working out, but water plays its part. Even sensitivity to insulin plays its part; dehydration causes higher insulin levels and inhibits fat burning. Because this contributes to type 2 diabetes, it's vital to keep your liquid intake at a good level.

Which Water Should I Choose?

Tap water is fine! If the water in your neighborhood is of high quality and tastes good, drink up! You'll save a small fortune over the course of the year if you go for tap water rather than bottled water. However, there are some natural springs that contain higher levels of minerals—mainly magnesium and calcium—and this can make it worth the money. Carbonated water is fine, too—even flavored ones—but definitely avoid water with any added sweetener. There are actually some brands of water that contain pure fructose, making them similar to soda. Some mineral waters (many of the more well-known brands) contain a lot of salt (sodium). In addition, in some varieties, the level of fluoride is unhealthily high; too much fluoride has been shown to increase the risk of osteoporosis and some forms of cancer. For both practical and economic reasons, you can carbonate and flavor your own water. A good trick is to add sliced cucumber, orange, or lemon to your water a few hours before serving; this gives the flavor without the calories. And these days, you can buy inexpensive machines to carbonate your water, giving you "sparkling water" at the push of a button.

Research Results

› Twenty-four overweight subjects drank either half a quart (half a liter) of water thirty minutes before breakfast or drank nothing at all. The meal was ad lib, and the subjects could eat as much as they wanted. The results showed that those who drank water ate 13 percent fewer calories than those who didn't have water (40).

› A large longitudinal study in which 173 overweight women aged 25–50 years were examined showed that a conscious increase in water intake to more than one quart (one liter) per day gave around a 4 ½ lb (2 kg) of weight loss over a year. Even the overall constitution improved (41).

› Seven men and seven women drank half a quart (500 ml) of water before their thermogenesis (heat production) was measured. As you might recall, this is one of the four factors of metabolism, and a small increase in thermogenesis over a long period of time can have a big effect. The increase in heat production was 100 KJ, equivalent to around 20 kcal. Around 40 percent of the energy went to increasing the temperature of the water from 71 F (22 C) to the body's temperature of 98.6 F (37 C). You can therefore assume that cold water from the refrigerator will increase heat production even further. For the men in the study, the increase in heat production gave an increase in fat burning, while for the women, it resulted in an increase in burning carbohydrates (42).

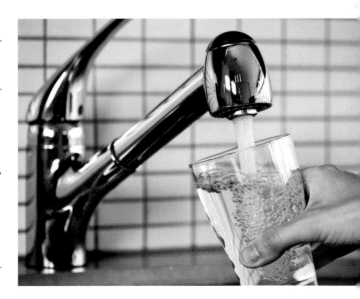

Red Wine

–Alcohol That Helps Metabolism

Personally, I enjoy drinking the odd glass of red wine, but it's very rare that I get drunk. The amount I do drink is sensible for both my health and weight, but you may be surprised to learn it's not only sensible, it can even be healthy. A moderate amount of red wine seems to be good for keeping your weight down (126, 127, 130). It seems strange because alcohol actually contains 7 kcal/gram, and the liver's metabolism pretty much ceases when we have alcohol in our blood (131). How, then, can a moderate intake of this calorie-rich liquid contribute to weight loss?

Of course, consuming large quantities of alcohol will make you fat because there are no compensatory effects in the world that can save us from thousands of extra calories, but drinking red wine in moderation can keep you trim in a few ways.

Alcohol's Effects

Alcohol reduces the secretion of parathormone (PTH), a hormone that inhibits fat burning and lowers resistance to insulin. Those who overproduce PTH gain weight (124). Alcohol also seems to increase the level of fat-burning hormones, such as glucagon and adiponectin (136). You can read more about this in the research results.

Alcohol releases dopamine, which stimulates the reward system in the brain. This is one of the reasons that so many people enjoy drinking alcohol. Dopamine is a strong neurotransmitter that gives us a feeling of well-being and purpose. Because we also get this feeling from sugar and fat, drinking a glass of wine can reduce cravings for candy, ice cream, cookies, and cake, making it easier to watch your weight. Maybe you also need less food to feel satisfied?

Sensitivity to insulin is also increased by alcohol (133, 135). So, when you have been drinking, your muscles and liver absorb more glucose, and your blood sugar and insulin levels decrease. As a result, it's easier to keep your weight steady. And, you're also protected against type 2 diabetes (134). This also explains, at least in part, why alcohol protects against heart disease, and it's also the reason why people with type 1 diabetes can experience dangerous swings in their blood sugar levels when they drink too much. There are many reports of cases in which diabetics have had near fatal drops in blood sugar when they drink. Perhaps this lowering of blood sugar is one of the reasons why so many people get the "munchies" and swing by a fast food joint on the way home from a night on the town.

Better Red than Sweet

Alcohol contains seven calories per gram, but around three of these disappear into heat while the alcohol is metabolized in the liver. This means that you don't actually gain as much weight from drinking alcohol as was once believed. However, watch out for calorie-laden drinks such as liqueur, cocktails, alcopops, sweet wines, and flavored (and sweetened) spirits. Creamy liqueurs such as Bailey's probably have the world record in empty calories. A ton of sugar and cream cancels out any positive effects from alcohol. Red wine, dry white wine, and beer, in that order, are the best forms of alcohol. Red wine has an incredibly high level of antioxidants, and the ORAC is between 2,500 and 5,000.

Some research shows that alcohol in the form of red wine is less fat-forming than other forms of alcohol (130). This may be because red wine contains resveratrol. In studies performed on animals, this molecule has been shown to increase fat burning (203), and in test tube studies on human fat cells, resveratrol has been shown to inhibit the maturation of proadipocytes (the early stages of normal fat cells) and the division of fat cells (319). Altogether, this should give fewer fat cells and make it easier to maintain your weight. However, remember that some red wines contain added sugar, so ask the liquor store staff. Hidden sugar is well known for keeping you from burning fat. You can also choose wines from France, where adding sugar to red wine is forbidden. If sorbic acid is present in the product (although this doesn't have to appear on the label), there is nearly always added sugar because sorbic acid is added to prevent the sugar from causing a second fermentation.

Research Results

> An American study looked at how alcohol consumption affected the weight of 19,220 healthy women over 39 years of age. The researchers thought that alcohol consumption would lead to an increase in weight during the thirteen years th at the study took place, but they found the complete opposite. Those who drank ½ to 1 oz (15–30 g) of alcohol per day, weighed the least of all. Teetotalers weighed the most and those who drank more than 1 oz (30 g) per day tended to weigh more than those who consumed moderate amounts (125).

> In a Dutch study, twenty healthy men aged 18–25 years drank either three cans of strong beer (a total of 1.4 oz [40 g] of alcohol) or three cans of light beer every day for three weeks. Those who drank strong beer had a higher level of adiponectin and glucagon than those who drank the light beer. This is interesting because both these hormones increase metabolism. Unsurprisingly, those who drank the strong beer also had a higher level of free fatty acids in their blood, which means that they should have a more effective metabolism than the light beer group (128).

> The same research group as above also wanted to study the effect of whiskey and asked eleven subjects of normal weight and eight subjects who were overweight to drink either half a cup (100 ml) of whiskey (1.1 oz [32 g] alcohol), or the same amount of water each day over the course of four weeks. Adiponectin increased by an average of 12.5 percent for those who drank whiskey, but those who had a normal weight also had an increase in their muscles' metabolizing capacity (129).

> In one study on diets, eighty-seven subjects were asked to ingest 1,500 kcal/day over the course of three months. Ten percent of the calories came either from grape juice or white wine. The calorie intake was the same, but those who drank wine lost an average of 10.4 lb (4.73 kg), and those who drank grape juice lost 8.3 lb (3.75 kg) (132).

So, the bottom line for alcohol is that it's beneficial to weight loss and helps us maintain our weight, but only when we keep to the recommended one or two glasses a day. More than this will give you an excess of energy and may be toxic. Unfortunately, there are many who just can't limit their alcohol consumption and will instead drink a bottle of wine at any opportunity. And unfortunately, consuming a small amount of alcohol a day is an easy way to become an alcoholic; as you become accustomed to the amount, you may find it becomes easy to drink more and more. It's estimated that there are more than 12 million alcoholics in the United States, and there are many more who binge drink. Such people should abstain from alcohol, so before you try out this shortcut, you may want to consider all the consequences carefully.

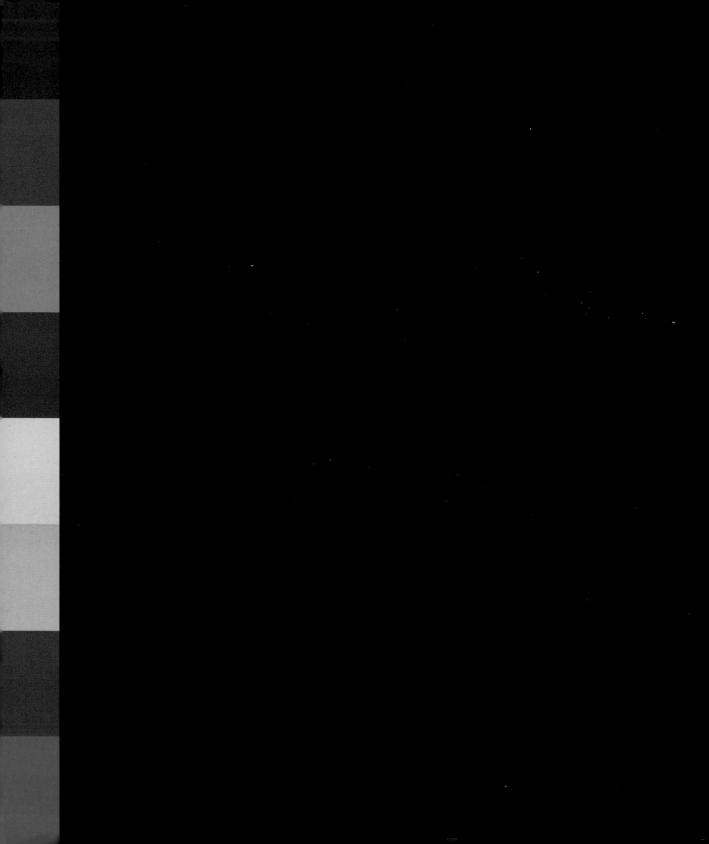

Spices That Boost Your Metabolism

26

The Chili Pepper

–A Warm Friend

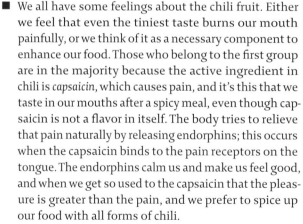

■ We all have some feelings about the chili fruit. Either we feel that even the tiniest taste burns our mouth painfully, or we think of it as a necessary component to enhance our food. Those who belong to the first group are in the majority because the active ingredient in chili is *capsaicin*, which causes pain, and it's this that we taste in our mouths after a spicy meal, even though capsaicin is not a flavor in itself. The body tries to relieve that pain naturally by releasing endorphins; this occurs when the capsaicin binds to the pain receptors on the tongue. The endorphins calm us and make us feel good, and when we get so used to the capsaicin that the pleasure is greater than the pain, and we prefer to spice up our food with all forms of chili.

In order to utilize capsaicin's benefits to our metabolism, it really helps to get used to it. You can start with a tiny drop of Tabasco and gradually increase the amount you use. When consumed through food, capsaicin is harmless; it's only if you eat it in its concentrated form (i.e., its pure chemical form), that it can cause harm. But pure capsaicin isn't sold to the average person, and is handled by chemical companies as hazardous goods. So be liberal with the spice in your food!

In Europe, the average daily intake of capsaicin is about 1.5 mg, whereas in India and Mexico it can be between 25-200 mg (294). Research shows that part of capsaicin's effect is dependent on its coming into contact with the stomach. Therefore, a supplement with chili/capsaicin is unlikely to be effective if it doesn't dissolve before reaching the small intestine (7). About 85 percent of capsaicin is absorbed in the gut, and a fatty meal allows for a more effective absorption because capsaicin is a fat-soluble substance. When it has been absorbed, it travels via the blood through the whole body and does its work here and there. One of the first signs of having eaten chili is an increase in your blood circulation.

How Does Capsaicin Work?

How does a strong spice increase your metabolism and contribute to weight loss? Your energy expenditure increases because the sympathetic nervous system is activated, counteracting the storing of fat. If you test the effect of capsaicin on fat, cells in a test tube, you can see that the fat cells don't absorb fat, but rather release it (14). In reality, this effect means that it's easier to burn the fat in your muscles and other organs. A consequence of an increased metabolism is that you give off heat, and when the body's core temperature rises, your appetite decreases. The burning sensation in the food also means that a lot of people pause more when eating and begin to feel full before they get a chance to overeat. Chili can, therefore, both increase your metabolism and reduce the amount you eat. In addition, it seems as if the energy intake will also be less at your next meal (5).

Research Results

Because different types of chili products have varying degrees of capsaicin, it's hard to do studies on its effects if you're not using pure capsaicin. But, it should never be ingested, (except in instances of research), because the risk of overdosing is high, and for some people, capsaicin can damage the nervous system, amongst other risks. In some studies, chili peppers have been used, but because we don't know exactly how strong they are, the exact effect is hard to evaluate. Nevertheless, here's a small overview of some of the studies of the effects of capsaicin/chili pepper.

> One of the earliest human studies on this subject took place in Japan and showed that 0.3 oz (10 g) of chili eaten after breakfast had an interesting effect. The chili increased both metabolism and fat burning, and the effect on fat burning was highest amongst those who ate breakfast with the highest fat content. With those who ate mainly carbohydrates, fat burning was increased, whereas the metabolizing of carbohydrates was reduced. This is interesting for those who do endurance training (10).

> Another Japanese study showed that chili mainly increases metabolism and reduces the appetite among those who eat fats. Metabolism doesn't get the same kickstart from chili if you eat a reduced-fat diet (17).

> A third Japanese study showed that chili peppers mainly increase the raised metabolism you get from a meal. At the same time, they can reduce the lowering of fat burning that takes place after we eat. Note that chili peppers only work if you eat them together with a meal. Capsaicin is actually fat soluble, and if there is no fat in the gut, then the absorption is negligible (11).

> A Dutch study showed that 4 ¾ oz (135 g) of capsaicin gave an increase in fat burning in the period following weight loss. Those who were given capsaicin burned 0.14 oz (4.2 g) of fat per hour during rest, as compared to those who got a placebo and burned 0.12 oz (3.5 g) per hour (6).

> A Japanese study showed that strong yellow curry increased the metabolism of women of an average weight. However, overweight women did not have the same experience. This could be due to the fact that a lot of excess weight is more insulating, so the body can't increase in temperature without the risk of overheating. This shows that capsaicin is probably best for people who have a few extra pounds to lose and want to avoid gaining weight (7). An alternative interpretation is that some people don't react as well to factors in their diet that can increase thermogenesis, and they therefore gain weight.

Good Sources of Capsaicin

- **Fresh chili pepper**
- **Dried chili pepper**
- **Unsweetened chili sauce (like Tabasco)**
- **Sambal oelek**
- **Strong curry powder**
- **Strong curry paste**
- **Piri piri**
- **Feferoni peppers**
- **Habanero**
- **Gochujang (Korean fermented chili paste)**

Bad Sources of Capsaicin

- **Sweet chili sauce (the sugar inhibits fat burning)**

Chili Pepper AND Caffeine

–One Plus One Is Three!

■ Sometimes a study will test a combination of a few substances, even if it's not as scientific as when substances are tested in isolation. Occasionally, two substances will work together in synergy, and the effect will be absolutely shocking. In this case, the effect was so impressive that it actually got its own shortcut in this book. Chili pepper and caffeine seem to give one another's effects a lift. Because capsaicin and caffeine are substances that normally appear in food, it is easy to apply this in real life.

How Do They Work Together?

The interesting thing is that both caffeine and capsaicin increase metabolism and fat burning, but they do so in slightly different ways. If you utilize both these substances at the same time, it's likely that they won't cancel each other out, but will rather enhance one another's effects. In addition, both caffeine and capsaicin are appetite suppressants, but with slightly different mechanisms. A really hot chili con carne followed by a few cups of black coffee should do the trick when it comes to burning fat and losing weight.

In a Canadian study, a small group ingested 200 mg of caffeine three times a day, about 0.85 oz (24 g) of chili pepper spread out over two main meals (lunch and dinner), and two snacks. Researchers then compared this group with a group that did not eat the chili pepper and instead drank decaffeinated coffee. Both groups got to eat as much as they wanted. The results showed that those who got capsaicin and caffeine greatly increased their metabolism and their appetite was reduced. When they compared the average difference in energy balance, it was around 1000 kcal/day (15). Other studies have shown similar, although slightly reduced, effects from the chili pepper alone (16).

Mustard
—For Increased Metabolism

Another strong spice that can increase heat production and fat burning is mustard (21). It's not as well researched as the chili pepper, but the strength it has seems to be similar to that of the chili pepper. The active substance in mustard is called allyl isothiocyanate; this is a sulfur-rich substance that gives mustard its heat. Mustard increases the release of norepinephrine, which in turn gets the metabolism going. In one early study, researchers showed that one teaspoon of mustard together with one teaspoon of chili sauce increased metabolism after a meal. Without spices, metabolism increased by 128 percent, and with spices it increased by 153 percent (21). Unfortunately, the design of the study means that we can't see how much of the effect was due to mustard and how much was attributed to the chili.

Which Mustard Should You Use?

A problem with mustard is that many varieties are almost always full of sugar and fat, and these obviously reduce the effect. You probably burn fewer calories from the mustard seeds than what you get through the sugar and oil; therefore, it's crucial to use mustard powder or French mustard when seasoning your food. Both of these products can work in dressings, but French mustard is probably more useful as an alternative to sweeter varieties.

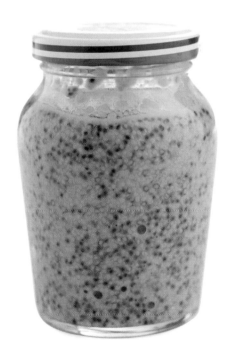

Ground Paprika
–The Mild Alternative

■ All types of paprika contain *capsinoids;* these are closely related to capsaicin, but lack the latter's burning sensation on the tongue and mucus membrane. Interestingly, capsinoids seem to be able to increase metabolism by binding to the same metabolism-enhancing receptors as capsaicin, but they don't cause the burning sensation. In an American study, capsinoids were shown to reduce weight among the test subjects; the biggest reduction was around the abdomen, which is interesting from a health perspective. It didn't seem as if metabolism was increased, but rather the rate of fat burning instead (9).

Burn Fat Without the Burn

When you compare paprika plants that lack the burning sensation (a known variety is called CH-19) with their spicier cousins, it seems as if both increase thermogenesis and, therefore, metabolism, regardless of their strength. Several studies show that CH-19 works just as well as the strong varieties to reduce the storage of fat. One difference between the two foods is that the stronger varieties temporarily raise your blood pressure and heart rate, which milder paprika doesn't do. This is important information if you are sensitive to spicy food, but still want the advantage of increasing your metabolism (12, 13).

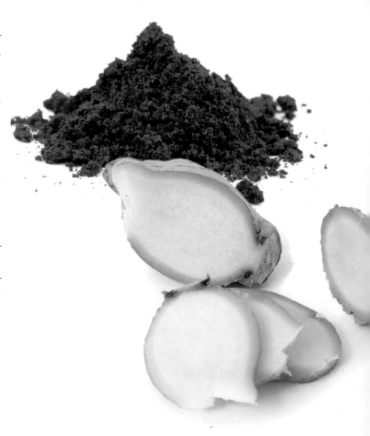

Ginger
–Spice Up Your Metabolism

Ginger is one of my favorite spices, and it's not just tasty, but also has positive effects on metabolism as well as on your health. Within alternative medicine, ginger is used in ayurvedic medicine to optimize metabolism and improve digestion, among other things.

Western research on ginger has mainly focused on its health benefits, but there are also studies that test ginger's effects on metabolism (19). Oxygen consumption among the test subjects increased—a clear sign of an increased metabolism (202). This effect is probably due to several substances present in ginger: among others, gingerol, shogaol, and zingerone, which can be compared to the capsaicin in chili peppers. Eating gingerol raises your body temperature, showing that the sympathetic nervous system is activated—just as with capsaicin. Studies in animals also show that the zingerones reduce fat storage in the fat cells (20).

It's possible that the combined effect of ginger and chilli peppers is even greater than when isolated, but at the moment, there are no comparative studies.

Another property of ginger that is of interest in regard to weight is that studies on animals have shown that ginger can inhibit the breakdown of fat in the small intestines. A Japanese study has shown that rats that are given ginger with a high-fat diet have lower blood fats and body weight than those that don't eat ginger, but get an otherwise identical diet. The reason for this is because the enzymes that break down fat in the rat's small intestine were inhibited, and the absorption of fat into the body was reduced (18).

What Form of Ginger Works?

The best way to eat ginger is undoubtedly fresh because it has the best taste, and the gingerol is intact. Chop, grate, or slice the ginger onto your food, but don't heat it too much. It can stand a bit of heat, such as light frying in a wok, but it shouldn't be heated to the point that it changes color. A great way to ingest the active substances in ginger is to add it to tea. You can flavor green tea with it, or simply make some ginger tea by pouring boiling water over a few ginger slices and letting it infuse for five minutes. It's a tasty caffeine free drink. Even dried, powdered ginger contains active ingredients and is an easy alternative when you have run out of the fresh stuff. Pickled ginger (like the variety you get with sushi) is fairly stripped of its goodness and has considerably lower levels of active ingredients than the fresh variety. Candied ginger is also not good because it's heavily sweetened, and the sugar will counteract all of its natural benefits.

Garlic
–Bad Breath, but Great Metabolism!

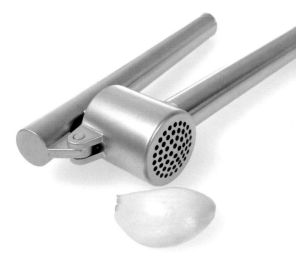

Garlic is mainly studied for its effect on the heart, and it has been shown to both lower blood lipids and reduce the tendency of blood platelets to clump together. So, garlic is effective for protecting against heart disease, and there is much that points to its having antibacterial and antiviral properties. This is why garlic is often used as a cold remedy. Garlic contains a lot of antioxidants and seems to increase your body's own production of antioxidants. The reason for this is its high sulfur content which is important if the body is to produce high levels of antioxidants. Many people believe that garlic can increase fat burning and metabolism, but unfortunately, this is one of the least studied shortcuts.

There is a lack of human studies, and we know that studies on rats don't always have the same results as they would have on humans. However, when it comes to rats, studies have shown that a diet containing 0.3 oz (8 g) of garlic powder per 2.2 lb (1 kg) of food over a period of twenty-eight days caused weight loss. When researchers looked at the reasons, it seemed that the amount of uncoupling proteins in the brown-fat tissue had increased. Put simply, this means that the rat's ability to convert fat to heat had increased (22). Another study examined the effect of allicin (one of the active ingredients in garlic) on weight gain in rats that were overfed. The result showed that the garlic extract greatly counteracted weight gain, while the rats that were given the same food without garlic quickly became fat (23).

When will we know the extent of the effect garlic might have on humans? First, it requires many more studies to be performed, but this is a shortcut in which it doesn't really matter if you take a chance. Garlic is incredibly healthy in so many other ways, and it's known to strengthen your immune system.

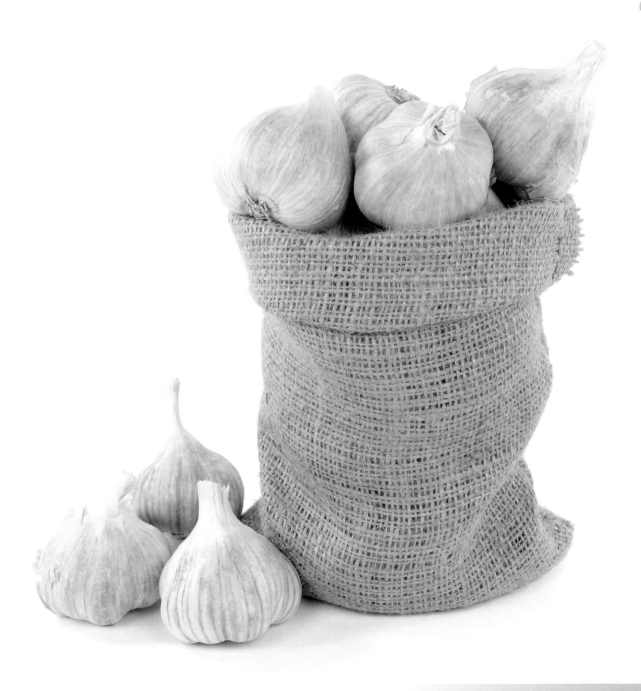

Cinnamon
–Lowers Blood Sugar

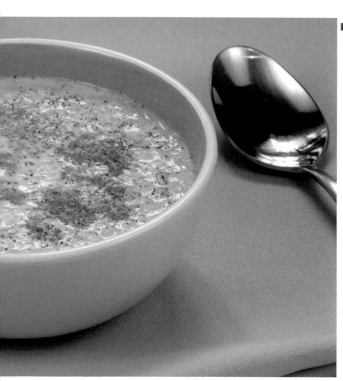

■ Cinnamon is a favorite spice for many people. It's used on porridge, in muesli, or over a fruit salad, and it would probably be used even more if people knew how healthy it really is.

Research has shown that cinnamon contains polyphenols. These shape the muscles to absorb glucose as it enters into the blood stream. In addition to working as an antioxidant, cinnamon helps your body keep the blood sugar in balance. It acts like an insulin mimic, increasing the muscles' ability to absorb glucose. Cinnamon can, therefore, help unlock the cells to glucose without the body having to secrete any insulin. Even the emptying of the stomach is affected by cinnamon; it simply slows down when cinnamon is added to the food you eat (35).

A meal containing cinnamon does not give the same increase in blood sugar as a meal without cinnamon. Therefore, when you include cinnamon in your food, the insulin levels will be kept on a more healthy level, allowing your body to burn fat. This is interesting because lower insulin levels mean less stored fat. It's pretty much impossible to get fat without insulin, and the lower levels of insulin you have, the more fat you're able to burn.

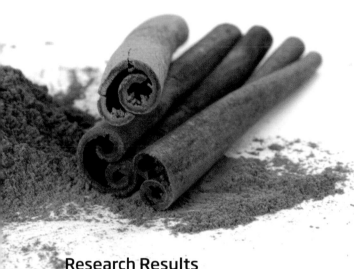

Research Results

There are several studies of cinnamon and its effects on blood sugar levels and fat burning. Here is a random selection.

› A study of eight healthy men of average weight showed that 0.1 oz (3 g) of cinnamon taken daily for two weeks lowered the fasting glucose (a term used to describe glucose levels before breakfast or after a longer period of fasting) levels by 13.1 percent as quickly as the day after the first dose. After two weeks, insulin levels were 27.1 percent lower in the cinnamon group compared to those who received a placebo (32).

› An American study of twenty-two people with early signs of type 2 diabetes showed that a daily supplement of the substances found in cinnamon (500 mg cinnamon extract, which is equal to 0.10 oz [3 g] cinnamon) had positive effects on both blood sugar and body constitution after a daily dose taken for twelve weeks. The fasting glucose sank by 8.4 percent, and body fat sank by 0.7 percent. The latter may not sound like much, but remember that it was only a two-week study, and only cinnamon distinguished the two groups. For a person weighing 220 lb (100 kg) with 40 percent body fat, reducing it to 39.3 percent means 1 ½ lb (0.7 kg) lost

simply by adding cinnamon. In addition, the cinnamon group increased their muscle mass by 1.1 percent (33).

› A British study of seven men of average weight showed that 1 tsp (5 g) of cinnamon a day lowered glucose by an average of 13 percent. An interesting observation is that cinnamon's effect lasted for more than twelve hours after it had been consumed. So, a dose at breakfast should last you the whole day (34).

› A study of fifteen women with PCOS (one of its symptoms is insulin resistance) showed that taking cinnamon extract daily over the course of eight weeks caused a clear improvement in insulin sensitivity (36).

› 79 type 2 diabetics were given cinnamon extract equivalent to 0.10 oz (3 g) of cinnamon daily (divided over three daily doses) over the span of four months. The fasting glucose sank on average by 10.3 percent, and it seemed to be more effective the higher the starting values were (37).

› The first study on cinnamon and blood sugar came in 2003. Sixty type 2 diabetics were given either a placebo or a certain amount of cinnamon each day for forty days. The amount of cinnamon was 0.03, 0.1, or 0.2 oz (1, 3, or 6 g) daily. Interestingly, all doses were effective. The fasting blood sugar levels sank by 18–29 percent, the LDL cholesterol was reduced by 7–27 percent, and the triglycerides fell by 23–30 percent. My interpretation is that 0.1 oz (3 grams) per day is the dose to aim for because the 0.2 oz (6 g) did not cause a significantly better effect. However, 0.03 oz (1 g) is better than nothing (38)!

How Should I Eat Cinnamon?

Take about a teaspoon of cinnamon each day in some form or another. It can be part of your breakfast, or you can sprinkle some in your tea or coffee. When you are preparing your drink, the active properties in cinnamon will dissolve and will provide flavor as well health benefits. Or you can just drop a teaspoon of cinnamon into the fresh coffee grounds when brewing in a coffee maker. You can even choose a cinnamon flavored tea because it has the same effect. Just use ground cinnamon, as it's difficult to get the polyphenols out of a cinnamon stick.

Fenugreek
–A Spice on the Way Up

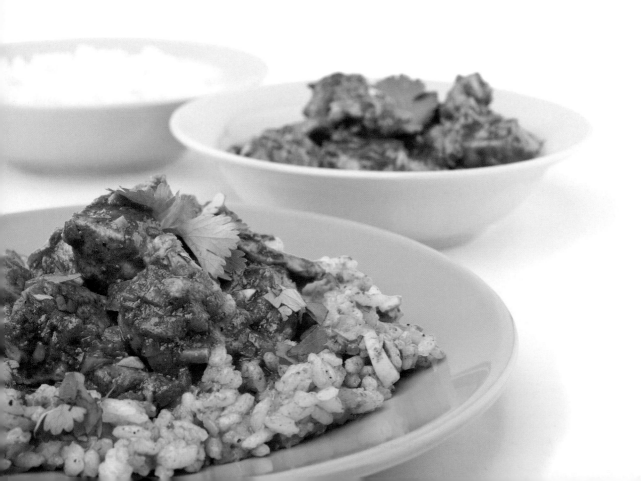

■ Surprisingly, fenugreek gets its own shortcut. Sure, we've read about other spices, such as chili pepper, ginger, cinnamon, and mustard, but how did fenugreek come into the picture? It's not something you hear much about. Unfortunately, this is mainly because studies on spices haven't been a particularly high priority. This may sound cynical, but it is probably due to the fact that there are no strong economic interests tied to this subject. It's far more lucrative to look at supplements or medicines, and had research on spices been a slightly higher priority, I'm sure there would have been many more shortcuts on the spice rack.

What's interesting to me is that many more spices are likely to be attributed with fat-burning properties in the future. Nearly every spice studied shows some potential. For example, researchers have looked at the effect of black pepper and its active ingredient *piperine* on rats, and they concluded that it has a similar effect to that of capsaicin (294).

Give Fenugreek an A+

However, back to fenugreek—a spice you probably don't have a ton of in the pantry. Most people don't even think they've seen it before, and are unsure about what form it takes. However, despite this, many of us actually eat it regularly because it is contained in curry. Indian food, in particular, is very rich in fenugreek. But, you can buy it separately and experiment with adding it to various dishes. Rice laced with fenugreek is a solid flavor combination, and bread baked with it is quite tasty (although you have to be careful to balance the amount because it's possible to affect the bread's taste and consistency). However, about 5 percent of fenugreek in the bread will go unnoticed (188).

Traditionally, fenugreek is used for Type 2 diabetes patients, but it's also used to stimulate milk production in mothers who breastfeed. It also seems to balance blood sugar and improve blood lipids among type 1 diabetics (187), a fact that is beneficial even for people who are perfectly healthy.

Research Results

❯ Twelve healthy men were given a daily supplement fenugreek extract, increasing in quantity over fourteen days from 0.588 mg to 1,176 mg. When the subjects consumed the higher amounts, they spontaneously ate 17.3 percent less fat than the control group, and their energy intake was 11.7 percent lower than the controls'. If this were translated to a daily intake of fenugreek over a longer period of time, the effect would be very large (186).

❯ In one study, researchers looked at the effect of two slices of bread with or without five percent fenugreek. The test subjects were all diabetic, and those who ate the bread laced with fenugreek had significantly lower blood sugar levels than those who did not eat it (188).

❯ It even seems as if the fibers in fenugreek are beneficial. In one study, the subjects were given either 0.4 g or 8 g of fiber from fenugreek in their breakfast, and they were later asked to eat until they were full at a lunch buffet. Those who consumed the highest fiber level automatically ate less for lunch. Obviously, this is beneficial to your metabolism (254).

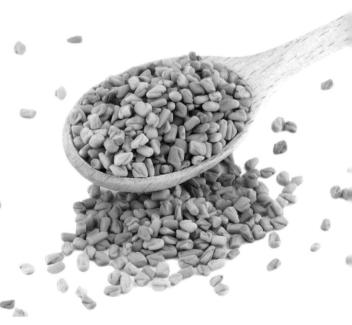

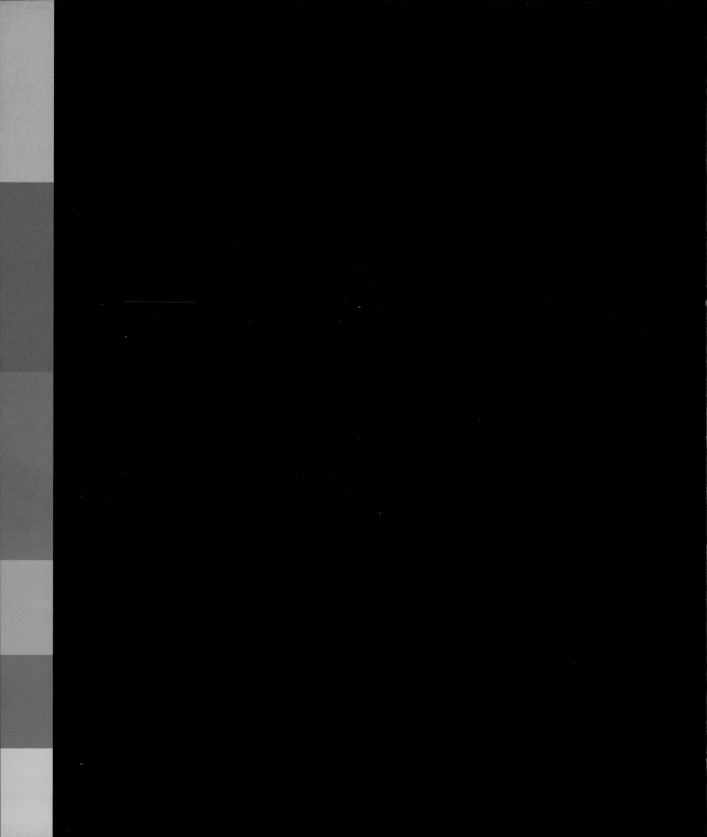

Nutrients, Hormones, and Other Bits and Pieces

Calcium

–A Great Surprise

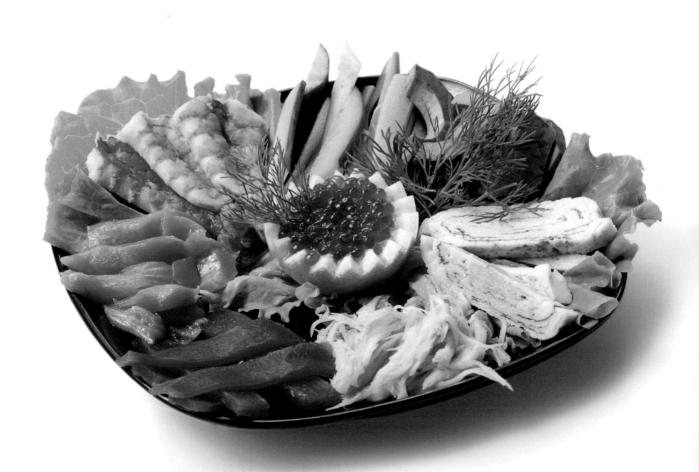

Sometimes the results of scientific studies can surprise you. One of the biggest surprises for me over the last few years was that calcium intake is linked to weight. Normal calcium plays a very important role in keeping weight steady. A review of five different scientific studies concluded that a supplement of 1,000 mg calcium a day over a period of four years could cause a weight loss of as much as 17.5 lb (8 kg). Another study showed that a 1,000 mg calcium supplement taken daily over the course of a year resulted in almost 11 lb (5 kg) of weight lost. This means calcium-rich food can be of even greater importance to keeping your weight down than was previously thought (96).

Why Is Calcium So Beneficial?

So, how can calcium reduce weight, and how does this occur? There seem to be several factors involved. Studies show several effects of calcium on body weight. First, it causes the fat cells to release more fat, which increases the potential for other cells—including the muscle cells—to burn fat. Calcium also decreases the uptake of fat to the fat cells, and produces a modest increase in body temperature, which leads to weight loss. Another possibility is that calcium seems to be a very weak natural Alli—a medicine that inhibits the breakdown of fat and its subsequent absorption in the bowels. Maybe you can take advantage of this and pop a calcium supplement during Thanksgiving dinner, dinner parties, and other calorie-laden events. With chocolate, added calcium can reduce the absorption of cocoa butter by 13 percent; this is likely because calcium raises the pH value in the bowels, and the enzymes that break down fat (lipases) can't function as effectively. All enzymes have a pH value at which they work best. As soon as the environment in the bowels is outside this optimal pH value, it reduces the ability of the lipases to break down fat, and more of this fat ends up in the toilet. Finally, it also seems that calcium is needed to regulate appetite. Those who suffer from a lack of calcium tend to eat more than they need (91).

Calcium in Food

Though calcium is most studied as a weight-loss aid in supplement form, it is, of course, just as effective to obtain it through the foods we eat. Some research shows that this is an even more effective method (295, 296). If you eat a calcium-rich diet, chances are you will lose weight.

In this shortcut, you will find two different lists with some calcium-rich foods. Remember, though, that some of them give a lot of energy, and that the amount of calories can be high in relation to how much calcium you get. Fish, shellfish, and vegetables are the most calcium-rich foods, and maybe this contributes to these foods keeping you in shape. Even low-fat dairy products have a lot of calcium per calorie.

Apart from the fact that calcium is good for keeping you fit, it also protects against osteoporosis and some forms of cancer. Women need around 800-1,200 mg, and men need 800-900 mg a day to avoid calcium deficiency. But, calcium can be more beneficial than just this. A few grams of it per day can be effective, and you can consume this amount by choosing calcium-rich foods and possibly taking a supplement.

Research Results

› A Canadian study of sixty-three overweight women showed that those who began with the lowest intake of calcium saw the greatest effect on their weight and body fat when they began taking a calcium and vitamin D supplement. Interestingly, the vitamin D was necessary for the calcium to reduce fat. The amount was 600 mg calcium and 5 micrograms of vitamin D taken as a supplement every day for fifteen weeks (74).

› An American study looked at the effects of calcium taken as a supplement versus a high intake of calcium-rich foods on fat burning and metabolism. The subjects were twenty-four women who were moderately overweight. They were given a diet that had a 500 kcal/day energy shortfall, and those with the highest intake of calcium had the highest level of fat burning (76).

› A longitudinal study that was carried out over a year-long period showed that the more calcium women ate, the less abdominal fat they had. The study was concerned with calcium present in food and not as supplements (90).

› It seems as if calcium from low-fat dairy products is the best way to kickstart weight loss and fat burning. In a study of 100 overweight women, subjects ate a daily diet with a 500 kcal/day deficiency for a period of eight weeks. They were divided into four groups and were given either 600 mg of calcium from mixed sources (group one); the same diet as group one but with 800 mg calcium taken as a supplement (group two); a dairy-rich diet with three portions of fat-free milk per day (group three); or a diet that contained three portions of calcium-enriched soy milk (group four). Group one lost 6.34 lb (2.87 kg) on average, group two 8.6 lb (3.89 kg), group three 9.76 lb (4.43 kg), and group four lost 7.63 lb (3.46 kg) on average. There seems to be something additional in milk that contributes to weight loss; my guess is that protein plays a large part (89).

The Right Amount from Supplements

If you take a supplement to get your daily dose of calcium, it's important that the tablet also contains magnesium and vitamin D (to make sure your body absorbs as much as possible from the calcium). The suggested amount is a tablet containing 500 mg calcium, 250 mg magnesium, and 5 micrograms of vitamin D, taken twice a day. Taking one in the morning and one in the evening is a good spread.

Foods Rich in Calcium

Milligram calcium per 3.5 oz of product

Cheese 28 % fat 740
Nettles 490
Whey cheese 8 % fat 340
Rosehip 310
Sweet almonds 265
Herring in tomato sauce 200

Soy flour 199
Sardines in oil 191
Hazelnuts 188
Sardines in tomato sauce 174
Frozen spinach 170
Dophilus 160
Dried figs 144
Rhubarb 140
Egg yolk 140
Frozen collard greens 136
Brown beans 135
Prawns 115
Perch 110
Skimmed milk, soured milk, yogurt 109

Milligram calcium per 1,000 kJ (around 240 kcal)
Note the incredibly high levels of calcium in vegetables in comparison to their energy content!

Nettles 1,960
Frozen spinach 1,700
Rhubarb 1,400
Frozen collard greens 910
Lettuce 810
Skimmed milk 680
Chives 640
Chinese cabbage 560
Semi-skimmed milk 540
Radishes 510
Cheese 28 % fat 475
Sauerkraut 465
Leeks 435
Lettuce 385
Cabbage 345
Blackcurrants 325
Cucumber 315
Perch 305
Frozen green beans 275
Frozen broccoli 275
Red cabbage 265
Canned tomatoes 260
Prawns 250

CLA
–The Multifaceted Metabolism- Boosting Pill

Toward the end of the '90s, the supplement CLA appeared on the market and was sold under various labels to great commercial success. It was launched because of several studies on rats that showed CLA could increase muscle mass while reducing fat at the same time. As if this weren't enough, it also seemed to reduce the risk of cancer in rats. Products flooded into the market, and shortly thereafter came several studies on humans. These studies showed that CLA did have an effect, but it was considerably less than the effect on rats, and so the flurry of interest surrounding CLA died down. In addition, several studies were published showing that for some people, ingesting CLA could result in undesirable side effects. The interest in the product sank even lower. Today, CLA has a small following, and products that have been researched less and have a lesser effect do better on the market. In this shortcut, my aim is to explain what CLA actually does and whom it can benefit.

Why Does CLA Burn Fat?

There are several reasons as to why CLA increases fat burning. Firstly, it seems as if CLA inhibits the enzymes that deal with the production of fat in the body. The use of fat as fuel, or fat burning, increases at the same time as heat production, and this raises the metabolism.

It also seems as if CLA prevents fat from entering the fat cells (173). One study found an usual effect: CLA tends to reduce fat on the legs and lower half of the body more than other parts (176). The reason for this is unknown.

Some studies show that CLA reduces appetite and increases the feeling of being full after a meal (179). It's possible that CLA can speed up the so-called *apoptosis* of fat cells while preventing the production of new ones (181). In simple terms, this means that more fat cells die and fewer are produced. If this is the case, CLA should give some people long-term effects that will remain visible long after they stop taking it.

CLA Builds Muscle

CLA is hardly the only supplement that can be attributed to burning fat; calcium, green tea extract, and chili peppers extract also do this. However, very few supplements share CLA's other benefits, such as increasing muscle mass. And more muscles equal better fat burning. As you know, muscles are active parts of the body, which burn fat simply by existing.

Research Results

› An intriguing study on rats showed that CLA (0.5 percent of the caloric intake over six months) significantly increased muscle mass. In addition, the ATP production in the mitochondria increased, which can be interpreted as a more effective muscular metabolism. At the same time, two important antioxidants produced by the body (*catalase* and *glutathione peroxidase*) increased–a sign of better protection against free radicals. Free radicals are molecules that lack an electron, making them highly reactive. They "steal" electrons from DNA, fats, proteins, and other molecules, which causes significant damage. Many serious health problems including diabetes type 2, cardiovascular disease, cancer, and premature aging, are related to high levels of free radicals (172).

› Another study of forty-eight men and women showed that taking 0.2 oz (6.4 g) of CLA a day for twelve weeks gave an average of 1.4 lb (0.64 kg) increase in muscle mass (182). Research also shows that you regain muscle mass lost during extreme dieting more quickly if you take CLA (180).

› In one study, fifty-five overweight post-menopausal women were given a supplement with either 0.3 oz (8 g) CLA or with the same amount of milk thistle seed oil for thirty-six weeks. The results showed that both oils reduced body fat, but did so in different ways. CLA reduced BMI and fat deposits, whereas milk thistle seed oil hardly affected BMI, but it reduced abdominal fat, lowered blood glucose levels, and increased muscle mass–a result typical of improved insulin sensitivity. It might be a good idea to take a combination of these oils to reduce the risk of insulin resistance (117).

› A meta-analysis (when researchers examine relevant studies on a subject and present an average of the results) showed that 0.1 oz (3.2 g) of CLA caused roughly a 3.5 oz (100 g) weight reduction per week. In total, the researchers went through eighteen studies and saw that weight reduction was linear for at least six months (175). A big drawback of this study was that it focused on weight rather than the total effect on the body's constitution. As we know, muscle mass increases, so in reality fat loss should be greater than 3.5 oz (100 g) per week.

› In one study, butter was enriched with CLA so that the level of CLA was increased tenfold. However, it had no positive effect on either body weight or anything else (184). My guess is that it was the high levels of long-chained fats in the butter that worked against CLA's properties.

What Problems Can Arise from CLA?

A worrying effect is that CLA seems to lower insulin sensitivity (174, 178). It's not exactly clear how this works, but one possibility is that large amounts of CLA are created in the cell membranes, and because they are trans fats, they have a slightly different structure from normal fats (known as *cis-fats*). They can change the properties of the cell membranes and make it hard for insulin to send its signal into the cell. The words "trans fat" can be frightening to some, but you should be aware that the trans fats in CLA are not the same as the synthetic trans fats that can be found in hydrogenated fats. These latter are feared because even a small amount of synthetic trans fats increases the risk of stroke, type 2 diabetes, and certain forms of cancer. Naturally occurring trans fats, such as the ones found in CLA, do not seem to have this effect. Humans have actually consumed natural trans fats throughout history. Millions of years ago, our forefathers ate meat from ruminant animals on the African savannah, and later on we kept animals for meat and milk (which also has a natural trans fat content).

However, a high intake of CLA can cause problems with insulin sensitivity, but there have also been longitudinal studies in which overweight subjects were given 0.1 oz (3.4 g) of CLA daily over the course two

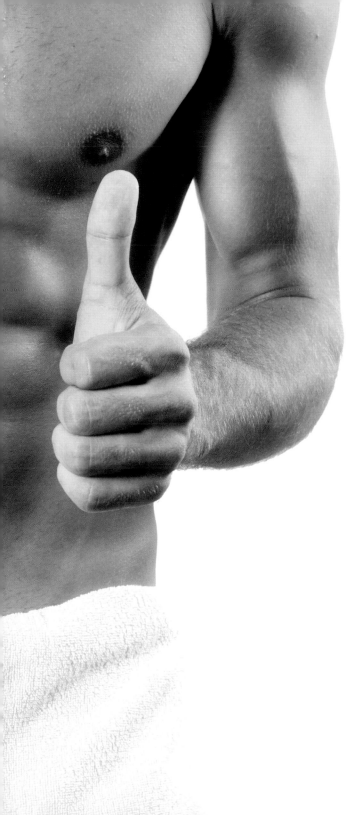

years, and no reduction in insulin sensitivity could be measured (177). In addition, total cholesterol was lowered as well as the bad cholesterol LDL, while the good cholesterol HDL remained unchanged. A Norwegian study has also shown that taking a daily dose of CLA for six months will not lower insulin sensitivity (183). And another study in which subjects took 0.2 oz (6 g) a day over the course of a year didn't show any changes in the glucose levels, either (185). So, clearly more research is needed!

Conclusions on CLA

My interpretation of CLA is that it works for some people for a limited amount of time, and it is one of the few supplements that can actually contribute to a better body constitution. Those who mainly benefit from CLA are those who work out a lot and want to get rid of any last few fatty bits to get that sixpack showing. The exercise will counteract any drawbacks of CLA, such as decreased blood lipids and insulin sensitivity, and these people will be content with losing just those extra couple of pounds of body fat. The small amount of muscle increase that CLA gives is also desirable for fitness fanatics.

If you are looking to lose many pounds, I believe CLA's effect is so small that it's not worth using. I also want to advise anyone with low sensitivity to insulin against CLA because there is a risk that it will worsen your condition. The same goes for those who have bad blood fats, inflammations, or liver failure because it's not clear how safe CLA is in these instances. If you do choose to use CLA, you should never take more than the stated dose and refrain from setting your expectations too high because CLA's effects are actually quite small. However, maybe you're only after getting a super sharp sixpack, in which case CLA's effects might be enough.

There is a study on rats showing that coconut fat can increase the effect of CLA (79). It's not clear if the combination works as well on humans, but you may as well try it if you plan on taking CLA (and as we know from earlier, coconut fat increases metabolism on its own).

Probiotics

–Train Your Intestinal Flora

■ Intestinal flora exists in your mouth, stomach, small intestine, and of course, your large intestine. Your intestinal flora, also known as *microbiota*, is sometimes referred to as your body´s largest organ, thanks to its many functions. In adults, the large intestine weighs from 4.5 to 6.5 lb (2 to 3 kg) and contains a large number of various bacterial strains. More and more research is showing that a balanced intestinal flora with the right combination of bacterial strains is vital for your gut to perform at its best (287). A classic example of what might occur if your intestinal flora becomes unbalanced is when you are infected by, for example, *Salmonella*—a particularly nasty bacteria that will knock everything else out if left to thrive. However, if you have good intestinal flora from the start, there are lots of bacteria that will kill the *Salmonella* and help you avoid an infection. Lots of people who have irritated guts will feel a lot better when they balance their intestinal flora with the right bacteria. New research also shows that the right microbiota improves your immune system, so taking a supplement of good bacteria can really work miracles. The latest research is focusing on microbiota's role when it comes to weight and metabolism.

I Have Strong Opinions

I may as well admit it from the start: I have strong opinions on the subject of probiotics—but they are good opinions! Since I started to understand the importance of our gut microbiota, I have become convinced that 90 percent of the people in the Western world should take a daily probiotic supplement. Originally, our diet was loaded with bacteria that entered our gut and colonized it. Evolutionarily speaking, we are built for consuming a diet full of bacteria, and it's only in modern times that the industrial handling of food and storage and preparation has eliminated this bacteria. Of course, we don't want to go back to the way food was handled in the Middle Ages, but we need to understand that we must add the right bacteria to food or take them as supplements. Personally, I have taken probiotics for the past five years, and I haven't had a proper cold for all that time. I also keep my weight steady better than I ever have, and I eat a diet based on the iso diet (but with some allowance for life's little pleasures). I work out regularly—not particularly hard or intensively— and I weigh as much today as I did when I was twenty

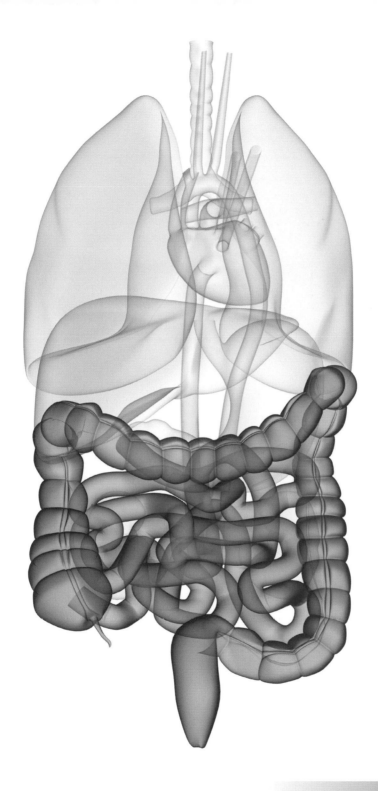

years old, so perhaps the bacteria have shown their qualities even in this respect.

How Can Our Intestinal Flora Affect Our Weight?

There are probably a range of factors that work together when it comes to probiotics' effect on weight (265). One of the more concrete factors is that probiotics can affect the breakdown of nutrients in the gut. Studies on animals, for example, show that a consumption of *Lactobacillus gasseri* inhibits the absorption of fat, which at least leads to slimmer rats (266). You can say that some of the fats *saponify* (get broken up and become water soluble) in the gut, and in this way avoid absorption and end up in the toilet.

Some bacteria have a higher metabolism than others and will simply steal some of the nutrients you eat before they reach the rest of your body. The release of so-called *gastric peptides* are affected by the intestinal flora, and these peptides affect energy balance

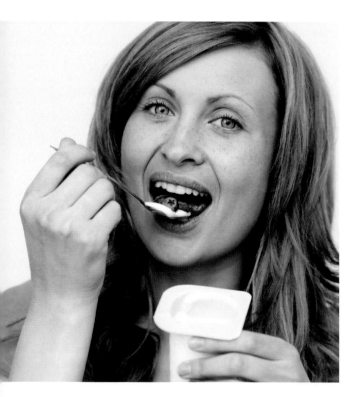

and storage of fat in different ways. The good strains of bacteria also inhibit the growth of the bad ones that produce endotoxins. These are mild poisons, which increase the level of inflammation in both the gut and the whole body, and we know that inflammations increase the body's tendency to store fat.

Another interesting angle on the subject is that some bacteria can produce fatty acids that stimulate fat burning. Animal studies have proven that *Lactobacillus plantarum* PL62 can produce CLA that actually seems to absorb into their bodies (268). The rats in the studies got thinner and had a more balanced blood sugar because CLA has the ability to increase your metabolism and muscle mass (see page 97). Even *Lactobacillus rhamnosus* PL60, which is usually found in the intestinal flora in humans, increased the CLA production in rats (270).

Unfortunately, it seems as if some strains can have the opposite effect, depending on their ability to break down fiber and produce short-chained fatty acids (274). These are generally good for us, but they also give us energy and have an effect on our energy balance. The result is that some strains help us lose weight while others can actually do the opposite. You can discover more about this in the shortcut on antibiotics.

The results you get from using probiotics also depend on what your intestinal flora was like to begin with.

Intestinal Flora Counts from the Start

When a child is born, it inherits a great deal of its intestinal flora from its mother. In the weeks after birth, the intestinal flora begins to establish itself properly, and the bacteria that the mother passes on makes a difference to the child. This is why Finnish researchers looked at what happened when they gave the expectant mother probiotics from four weeks before her due date until six months after giving birth. The results showed that probiotics (*Lactobacillus rhamnosus*) supplement protected against weight gain, but that this protection was reduced as more time passed and the probiotics were no longer being given (261). In my opinion, this is why everyone should take probiotics throughout their lives.

Another study showed that the risk of gestational diabetes was drastically reduced when expectant mothers were given *Lactobacillus rhamnosus* GG and

Bifidobacterium lactis Bb12 (264). Only 13 percent of women who received probiotics were affected by diabetes during their pregnancy, as opposed to the 36 percent who were given a placebo. In addition, the probiotics reduced the risk for unhealthily large babies. Mothers who have diabetes have higher insulin levels, resulting in quicker growth of the fetus. Babies that are unnaturally large at birth run a higher risk of being overweight and having metabolic disorders later in life; this is why taking probiotics when pregnant can be seen as a cheap and safe strategy to safeguard against future health problems for your children. Research has even shown that an imbalanced intestinal flora in children is strongly linked to future weight problems (269).

Research Results

› Eighty-seven subjects were given either 200 ml sour milk every day with a bacteria culture based on *Lactobacillus gasseri* or sour milk without any bacteria. The study continued for twelve weeks, and those who were given probiotics lost about 5 percent more belly fat. The total weight loss was 1.4 percent, and BMI was reduced by 1.5 percent; this might not sound like a lot, but remember that the individuals were fairly heavy, so we're talking about over two pounds lost simply by taking a healthy supplement. Probiotics are something you should eat all year round throughout your lifetime. Had they had continued the study for another year, maybe the subjects would have lost up to ten pounds (262).

Can Antibiotics Make You Fat?

The word antibiotic comes from the Greek, just like the word probiotic. Whereas probiotic means "for life," antibiotic means "against life." If probiotics make us thin, shouldn't antibiotics have the opposite effect? The question might seem naïve and simple, but it is highly relevant. Antibiotics have a wide reaching effect on a large number of bacteria in your microbiota; when you finish a course of antibiotics, your flora is highly affected, and many of the good bacteria that help with weight are gone. Also, the level of less desirable bacteria strains can increase dramatically.

As I have mentioned previously, certain strains of bacteria help keep our weight healthy, whereas others stimulate weight gain. So, altering the balance with antibiotics can have far-reaching consequences. The reason why some strains of bacteria can stimulate weight gain is that they are more effective in breaking down nutrients in the small intestine, so the absorption of calories is even greater. If you increase from 90 to 95 percent in the absorption of nutrients, it means 100-103 extra kcal per day, which is equal to roughly 11-15 lb (5-7 kg) of body fat.

A good example of how this can go wrong is when patients suffering from myocarditis (inflammation of the heart muscle) receive vancomycin and gentamicin, which eradicate most of the bacteria in the body. However, one specific strain of bacteria is resistant to these antibiotics, and it takes over the intestine and creates a more effective absorption of nutrients. One study measured the BMI of patients one month before their hospital stay and a year after they had left the hospital. Nearly everyone who had received this combination of antibiotics had a BMI that was more than 10 percent higher when the study ended (263). Therefore, the advice is to be careful with antibiotics if you want to keep your weight healthy.

How Do I Know Which Bacteria Are Good for Me?

This is not an easy question to answer, but there are some basic rules. Of course, the best evidence for the effects of probiotics is to test a specific strain to see that it has actually caused weight loss.

Bacteria are usually divided into several breeds: firmicutes and bacteroidetes (271). Overweight people have a higher level of firmicutes and a lower amount of bacteroidetes (272), and there is reason to believe that an adjustment of the intestinal flora could lead to weight loss. Even those with type 2 diabetes have a higher amount of firmicutes at the cost of bacteroidetes, so sensitivity to insulin is probably a central mechanism in this context (273). When it comes to probiotics, it's hard for the average person to put together the perfect product for weight loss when it comes to probiotics. My advice is, therefore, to choose commercially available products that are specific to weight loss, or alternatively, search for strains that you know have been tested (e.g., *Lactobacillus gasseri* and *Lactobacillus rhamnosus*).

The Thyroid Gland

–Keeps Your Metabolism Going

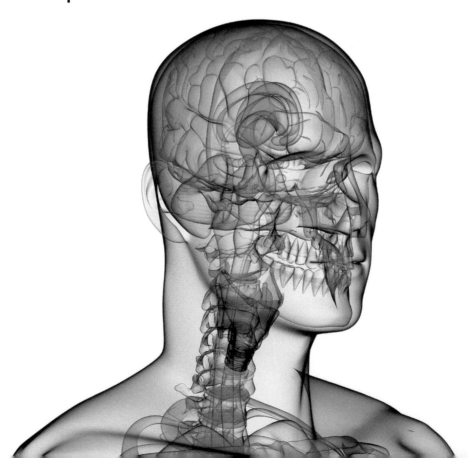

■ The thyroid gland is a small organ that sits at the front of the windpipe between the chest and the chin. Despite its diminutive size, the thyroid is very important because it produces, stores, and releases T3—a hormone that is strongly linked to metabolism. It has become more common to have slightly lower levels of T3; unfortunately, this doesn't just affect metabolism, but also the quality of life. We don't know why many people now have less T3, but it could be related to better methods of diagnosing the problem. The reasons for a deficiency can vary from an autoimmune reaction to surgical removal of all or part of the thyroid. There are also theories that long-term stress can lower the thyroid's production of T3. It's not easy to know if you suffer from hypothyroidism, as it is called, and only a visit to the doctor can discover this, but this is easily done and hypothyroidism is treatable. If you have some of the symptoms below, I suggest that you have a blood test done to check levels of T3:

- Depression
- Muscle cramps
- Brittle nails and hair
- A lowered production of sweat
- Weight gain and water retention
- Constipation
- Lowered heart rate
- Fatigue
- Brittle bones
- Memory loss
- Muscle weakness
- Myxedema (a collection of homogenous and gelatinous substances in the connective tissue that causes swelling)

Avoid Iodine Deficiency

Real hypothyroidism affects one to three percent of the population in the western world, but many more may have minor deficiencies and may suffer mild symptoms (such as a lower metabolism) without actually being considered ill. It's possible that a diet lacking in iodine can cause an underproduction of T3 because iodine is one of the building blocks of this hormone. Even a high intake of nitrate (present in many vegetables) can inhibit the absorption of iodine. This is why a strict vegan diet that doesn't allow for fish or shellfish can cause problems. Vegan women have an increased risk for giving birth to babies with a T3 deficiency (275).

To ensure that you don't experience a deficiency of T3 through keeping an unhealthy diet, you need to vary your food. T3 consists of the amino acid *tyrosine* and a number of iodine atoms (T3 has three and T4 has four), and if there is a deficiency, it is normally iodine that is lacking. The daily requirement for adults is 150 micrograms a day. In most Western countries, salt is enriched with iodine, and in my opinion, you should always choose this type.

Food with Iodine

- Iodine-enriched salt
- Fish
- Shellfish
- Algae
- Dairy products
- Eggs

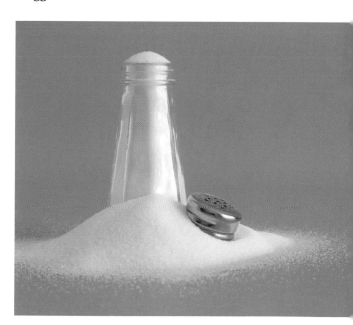

Testosterone

–A Male Shortcut?

■ Despite its being known as "the male hormone," both men and women have testosterone in their blood. However, men have about 10 times as much testosterone as women do, and women are much more sensitive to it. Nevertheless, the hormone is necessary for both sexes.

Women produce testosterone in their ovaries, whereas men produce it in their testes, and both sexes produce a small amount in the adrenal glands. There are also huge differences among individuals, giving some women higher levels of testosterone than some men. This is not considered abnormal. The studies in this chapter have almost all been done on men, so I'm sorry if it's not clear how women can achieve the same effect with this shortcut.

What Does Testosterone Do?

We tend to differentiate between testosterone's *anabolic* properties (which means that it builds muscle and bone) and its *androgen* properties (also known as masculinity). The latter is the development of the male sex organ, a deeper voice, and facial hair. For adults, testosterone is vital for health because it protects against heart disease and keeps body fat low—although sometimes it's hard to know which is the chicken and which is the egg because belly fat causes a lower secretion of testosterone and low testosterone causes belly fat. You can see it as a vicious cycle, and it is metabolic syndrome that's the real culprit. When you increase levels of testosterone in men with metabolic syndrome, the effect on weight can be dramatic.

There is a case of a man who had a testosterone level of 5.0 nmol/liter blood (normal levels are 12.0–33.0 nmol/liter). He had been given injections of testosterone to normalize his blood levels, and after sixteen weeks, he lost 110 lb (50 kg) (280).

Because testosterone builds muscle, the overall change in his body must have been very dramatic. To get rid of unwanted fat around the stomach, one strategy is to raise testosterone keep in shape this way. Testosterone's muscle building properties also make long-term fat burning easier because muscles keeps metabolism high. With older people, it also seems that testosterone plays a role in sensitivity to insulin and the regulating of blood sugar (279).

Metabolic Syndrome

Metabolic syndrome is a generic name for many related illnesses, and it causes (and is caused by!) insulin resistance (even type 2 diabetes), high blood pressure, obesity (especially belly fat), and a worsening of blood lipids.

How Do You Increase Testosterone?

It's only when you have a noticeable lack of testosterone that you should take testosterone-based medication. For healthy people, there are several simple things you can do to increase your level of testosterone.

Sleep well: Sleep, especially REM sleep, is important for the release of testosterone (281).

Weight training: Lifting weights gives a fairly quick increase in the release of testosterone and can be seen as the body adapting its need to build and repair muscle (282). Too much exercise, however, can lower testosterone and raise cortisol, so be careful to avoid this.

Eat properly: food made with quality ingredients with low GI, lots of antioxidants, and a relatively high intake of fats (40-50 percent of your total energy intake), but without trans fats, it is the recipe for a testosterone-raising dietary plan.

Check your zinc levels: Low zinc levels will inhibit the release of testosterone.

Have sex and/or think about sex: Both these activities increase the release of testosterone.

Avoid licorice: Interestingly enough, eating licorice can lower testosterone levels in the blood by about 25 percent for both men (284) and women (283).

Don't stress too much: It lowers testosterone and raises cortisol.

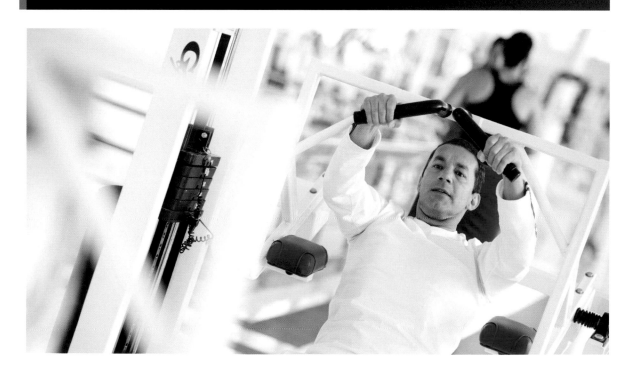

Vitamin D
–Crucial for Fat Burning

■ Vitamin D is a substance that has received a lot of attention in recent years. It's slowly dawning on us how incredibly important it is to our health. We have known for a long time that vitamin D strengthens our bones and, therefore, can protect against osteoporosis. New studies also show that it protects against many forms of cancer, autoimmune diseases, depression, heart disease, and type 2 diabetes.

Even your immune system is affected by the level of vitamin D in the blood. This can be one of the reasons why we are more likely to get a cold during the darker months of the year. Sunlight promotes the production of vitamin D in the skin, and many believe that our immune system's T cells need vitamin D to mature and do their job.

This vitamin also makes a difference in our shape. The reduced insulin sensitivity that affects those with low vitamin D levels makes it much more difficult to burn fat. As you remember, low insulin sensitivity is linked to increased insulin levels, and insulin is a hormone that stores fat. A Spanish study of 102 children aged 9-13 years showed that those who had the lowest levels of vitamin D in the blood also had the highest BMI and body fat (72). Another study showed that those with the best amount of vitamin D had the highest heat levels after they had eaten (76). The higher this is, the less likely your meals are to be stored as fat.

Does Vitamin D Kill Fat Cells?

Yet another interesting theory on why vitamin D seems to contribute to weight loss is that it's possible that it can reduce the number of fat cells in the body. Previously, researchers believed we had a fixed number of fat cells that hardly changed throughout our lives, but we now know this is not the case. Fat cells *can* increase in number, especially during childhood and pregnancy, but also when there is a need—such as when weight has increased to such a level that there is not enough space to store fat in the existing fat cells. On the other hand, the number of fat cells can be reduced when you lose weight and no longer need them. This process is known as *apoptosis* and can be described as the cell "committing suicide." Exactly what signals stimulate apoptosis in the fat cells is not clear, but a test tube study has shown that vitamin D actually causes it (73). We can only speculate

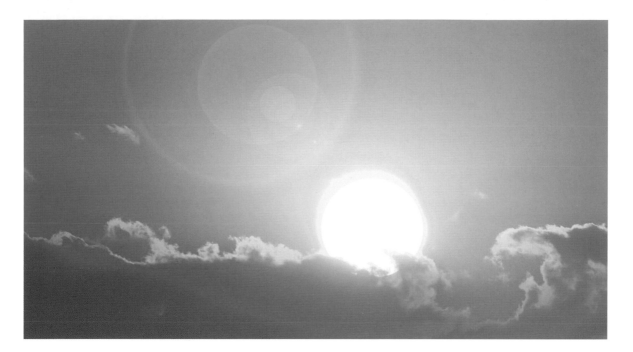

as to why this mechanism exists, but it seems logical that sunlight (and therefore vitamin D) is connected to warmth and a better chance of survival. When the temperature is warm, the need to store fat is reduced, and perhaps even the number of fat cells diminishes.

Metabolism and Calcium

On page 30, you can read about calcium's role in burning fat and controlling weight. Now, research shows that vitamin D is needed for calcium supplements to aid weight loss (74). This was fairly expected because vitamin D increases the absorption of calcium in the intestines where it can then enter the body and affect the fat cells.

Fat Muscles

Vitamin D also makes your muscles feel good. It seems that it is linked to muscle strength and balance. Many studies show that older people with a good level of vitamin D have stronger muscles and don't fall over as those with lower levels of vitamin D do. (78).

Even the muscles' fat storage is affected by vitamin D. If the muscles store fat because you are exercising a lot and it's required for fuel, then all is well. If they store fat because of overeating, a lack of exercise, or a lack of vitamin D, then this is less positive. Storage of intramuscular fat (fat stored in the muscles) is associated with insulin resistance and is one of the reasons why vitamin D is associated with type 2 diabetes. One study of women of average weight showed that those who had the lowest levels of vitamin D in the blood had the most fat marbled through their muscles (77). This is known as muscle adiposity, which can be described as muscle obesity. Even if the subcutaneous fat is not too obvious, you can still be "fat" inside your muscles.

Sources of Vitamin D

- Sunlight
- Egg yolks
- Margarine
- Dairy products
- Liver
- Dietary supplements

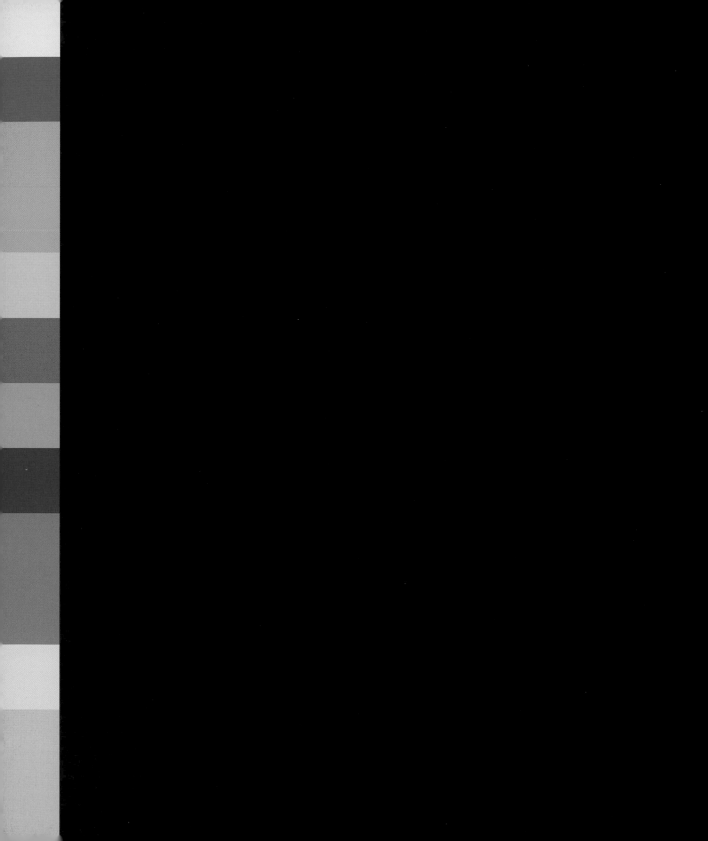

Feel Great and Increase Your Metabolism

A Morning Walk

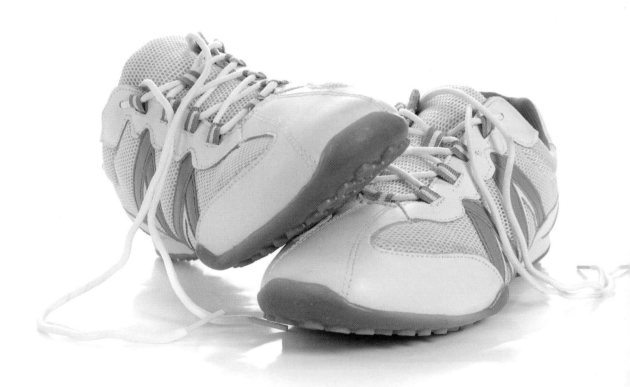

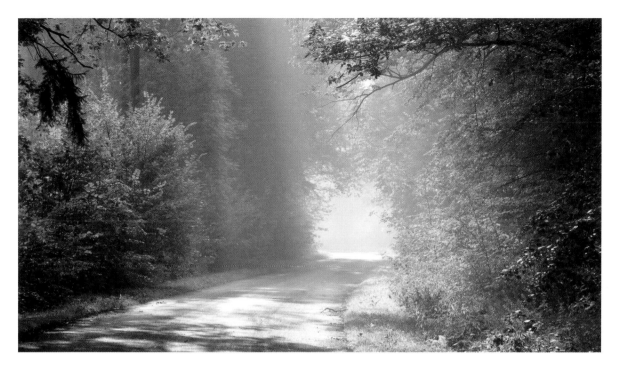

When you have just woken up, the hormonal environment in your body is almost perfect for fat burning. Insulin levels are low, and the effect of the night's release of growth hormone remains. As growth hormone is one of the body's most avid fat burning hormones—this is very good to know! Even other hormones that have a metabolizing effect, such as glucagon, are raised when you wake up. This is all because you haven't eaten anything for several hours.

The reason why you have the energy to exercise on an empty stomach is that the reserve of blood sugar in the liver is released, and in this way, you get enough blood sugar for an hour-long walk. In addition, you have some ketones that complement the blood sugar as brain fuel. At the same time, the fat cells are wide open and releasing fatty acids, which you can burn while working your muscles.

However, it's important that you don't exercise too hard before breakfast as atrophy of the muscles seems to increase (at about 65 percent of your maximum aerobic capacity). Therefore, stick to power-walking or light jogging.

Research Results

> In a Canadian study of eight young men, researchers examined how many grams of fat were consumed during an exercise session that required 400 kcal to complete. They used about 0.6 oz (17 g) of fat on an empty stomach before breakfast and about 0.4 oz (11 g) when they exercised after breakfast. That's a whole 50 percent more fat burning before breakfast (28).

> An American study examined if there was a difference between fit and unfit people in relation to how fat burning was affected by exercising before breakfast. Both the fit and unfit people had an improved rate of fat burning (29).

> One study showed that the heart rate is slightly higher when you work out before breakfast (30). The reason for this is that fat requires about 10 percent more oxygen than carbohydrates for each kcal that is extracted. A higher rate of fat burning therefore means a higher heart rate and more rapid breathing. It is, therefore, a slightly tougher form of exercise, especially because you don't have any blood sugar that can tell the brain that the energy supply is good.

Weight Training

■ Many of those who work out at the gym use both machines that aid fat burning and those that are more suited to purely strengthening the muscles. Even regular cardio sessions are often combined with a few weights, and the question that often arises is which should you do first—resistance training or cardio? However you look at the various components, exercise will give you results, but it's likely that fat burning and muscle building will be more effective if you do weights first and cardio last. One reason for this is that the general energy levels are greatest at the beginning of your workout, and weight training demands more power and energy. The fat-burning phase is often easier to get through on sheer determination because it's usually not as mentally taxing or particularly strenuous. Purely physiologically, your muscles primarily use *glycogen* (stored carbohydrates) when resistance-training and a combination of fat and glycogen when doing cardio. When the glycogen deposits reduce, which they will do quite quickly during resistance training, you become tired. Glycogen is stored in rather limited quantities in our muscles, so after an hour's resistance training, the stores are quite small. If you then go and stand on the treadmill or do some spinning, a larger part of the energy you use will come from fat. Had you done cardio first, the glycogen deposits would have run out and the resistance training would have suffered.

What Does this Mean from a Practical Point of View?

As your resistance training will go better due to larger levels of glycogen and fast fuel for your muscles, your muscles will develop better. In combination with the fact that this burns fat more effectively, your body's constitution will vastly improve. The more explosive resistance training you can manage, the better it is. Explosive training releases hormones such as growth hormones and testosterone in higher levels, which are involved in both fat burning and muscle building.

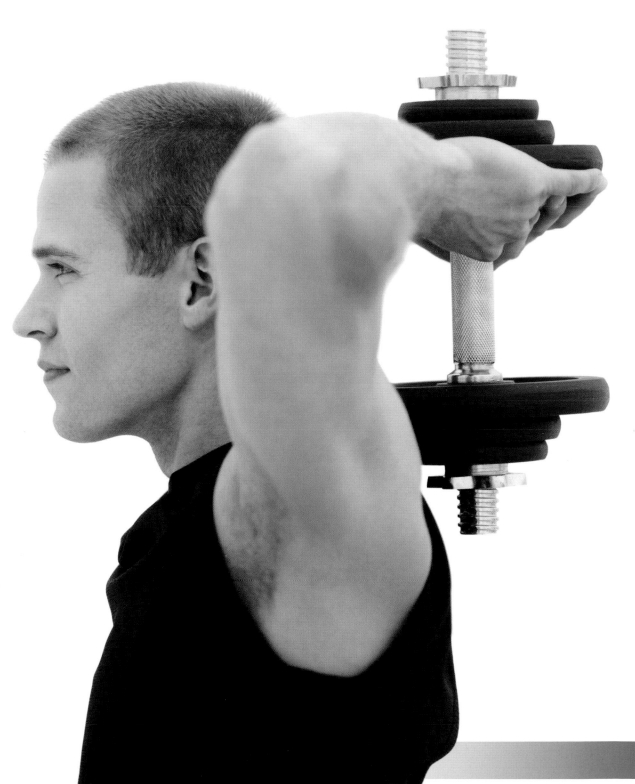

Fitness Equals Fat Burning

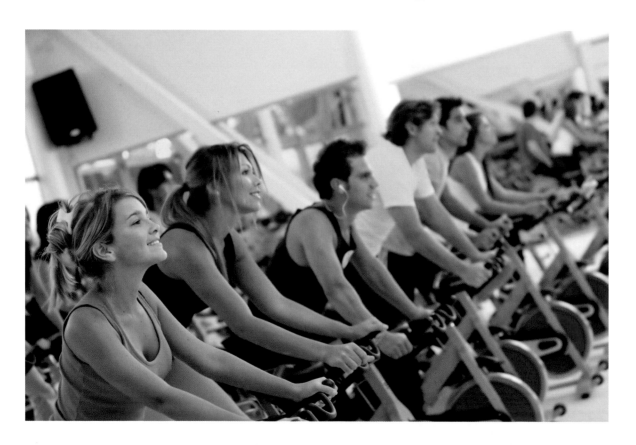

■ In theory, there's a very easy way to increase your fat burning—get fit! In practice, however, it's not always so easy, but it doesn't have to be hard! It does, however, it does require a degree of knowledge. You can make getting fit easy for yourself and, for example, start jogging. Much points to the fact that interval training is best if you want to see noticeable results in your fitness level, but simply jogging for half an hour three times a week is enough to significantly increase your fitness level. Make sure to remember that fitness needs to be maintained. Of course, it returns quickly if you've been fit in the past, but you really need to exercise a few times a week. If it's too cold to power-walk or jog, my advice is to find pleasant indoor activities that get you breathing heavily and your pulse going. Spinning, indoor sports, running on the treadmill, badminton, dance, and aerobics are all good examples of fitness-improving activities.

What Happens When Your Fitness Level Improves?

Essentially, you can say that the body becomes more effective at burning fat the more fit you are. Exercise causes a larger energy expenditure and oxygen consumption, and a large portion of this energy always comes from fat. Because we have large fat deposits, the use of fat for fuel increases once the body adapts to demanding forms of exercise. Fat is released from the fat cells, and there is a greater absorption of fat into the muscle cells' mitochondria. This is how a hazelnut can transform into a few running strides, or a square of chocolate into some dance moves. Chemical energy is simply transformed into movement energy, and suddenly the fat is burned off. The last thing necessary for fat to be metabolized is that the mitochondria has to have enough of the enzymes that steer this process. The quantity of these enzymes (beta oxidation) increases with your fitness level. In addition, some fat is stored in the muscles; this increases when you do a lot of endurance training and becomes an easily accessed source of energy. It seems that a good fitness level reduces the fat cells' ability to store fat and increases the muscles' fat storage. This isn't just functional—it also improves your physique.

What Do I Do if I'm Lazy?

If you are starting from a lower fitness level, even small things can make a difference. Many people believe that fitness can only be achieved through extreme exercise sessions, but nothing could be further from the truth. I would like to introduce the term *microtraining* into your vocabulary. Microtraining means always choosing the most difficult alternative. If you lose your breath when taking the stairs for a few flights, then this is just what you need to do. The results soon become quite evident. After a few weeks of regular stair-climbing, you won't be out of breath—proof that your effort has paid off! Your ability to absorb oxygen will improve, and this translates into a better fitness level and improved fat burning. Obviously, this is especially effective when exercising, but even at rest, you will burn more grams of fat per hour than you did before.

Microtraining can be applied in any situation imaginable. You're the only one who knows your daily routine and how micro training can be applied to it. It could be a slow jog to the bus, or stepping off the subway a few stops early on your morning commute. Parking the car a few blocks away or adding an obligatory twenty-minute walk during your lunch break will improve and/or maintain your fitness level. Other positive effects of microtraining are increased insulin sensitivity and actually increasing your metabolism the next time you exercise.

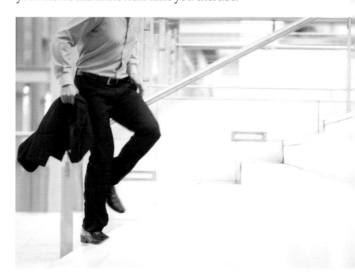

Walk Off Your Meal

■ Personally, I try to walk off what I've eaten whenever I can. This simply means that I'll take a walk after my meal; it doesn't need to be more than half an hour (which most people can squeeze into a lunch hour). What's the point of this? Well, your muscles will start to work, meaning they'll need more fuel in the form of carbohydrates. They can then absorb blood sugar without needing insulin to do so, and this in turn leads to lower insulin levels. As insulin inhibits fat burning, you can say that physical activity is the same as pressing the start button on fat burning.

How long should you walk for if you want to get the effects of lowered blood sugar and reduced insulin? Five minutes is, of course, better than nothing, but studies have never measured the effect of anything shorter than fifteen minutes. One study showed that even a slow-paced walk of fifteen-minutes' duration gave a measurable effect. Forty minutes gave, as expected, an even bigger reduction (191), so every step counts.

Metabolism Increases after a Meal

As you read at the start of the book, body temperature rises after a meal, and the more it rises, the more fuel for the fire the body has. From a fat-burning perspective, it's positive that the so-called mealtime-induced thermogenesis is high, and the truth is that it rises even higher when you gently exercise directly eating. This is why a walk after a meal increases metabolism (317). That you avoid sugar spikes at the same time is just a bonus for your health! High blood sugar tends to bind to the body's proteins and speed up signs of aging, and it contributes to illnesses such as heart disease, type 2 diabetes, and dementia. Don't get stuck in a lunch coma: Get of going in the walk of life!

> **Thirty minutes of fast walking after lunch five times a week will give you better insulin sensitivity and, over the year, 130 hours of exercise. You use up around 300 kcal per hour; after a year, that's 39,000 kcal, which is equivalent to about 12 lb (5.5 kg) of body fat.**

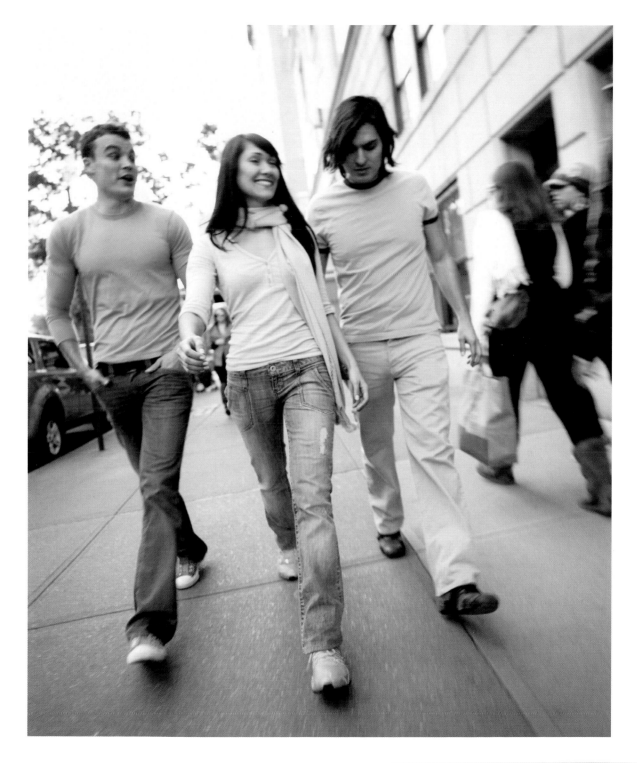

44

Sunshine Helps

◾ Sunshine provides us with UV rays, but too much exposure can damage our skin cells, resulting in increased risk for skin cancer, wrinkles, and other damage.

However, too little sun is equally damaging to our health. Sunshine is a must in order for our bodies—or more specifically, our skin—to create vitamin D. Vitamin D protects us against a whole host of health problems and illnesses: brittle bones, type 2 diabetes, cancer, heart disease, lowered immunity, neurological problems, and autoimmune diseases (see page 108). As if that weren't enough, a lack of vitamin D causes insulin resistance and weight gain. Research shows that the more vitamin D you have in the blood, the less body fat you have (120-122). This means that the lower the vitamin D levels, the more you weigh on average.

Melanocortin Metabolizes and Burns Fat

When UV rays reach the skin, the body creates more *eumelanin* to protect itself; eumelanin is what causes the dark color in the skin when we tan. In order for eumelanin to be produced, the body uses a type of hormone called *melanocortin*. These hormones make us tan, but they also increase fat burning and decrease our appetite (304). On a purely evolutionary level, it's smart for the body to reduce the fat deposits when the weather is warm; this way, you won't drag around unnecessary weight and become slow and vulnerable. In addition, this decreases the risk for heat stroke.

Melanocortin works by reducing the amount of calcium in our fat cells, which leads to an increase in fat burning (298). Studies on animals also show that the sun, via an increase in melanocortin, can actually increase metabolism. One reason for this is that the amount of UCP (a type of protein that converts fat to heat) increases in the cells(299-302).

Another is that melanocortin seems to stimulate the release of the thyroid hormone T3 (303), which is a hormone that we know stimulates both metabolism and fat burning.

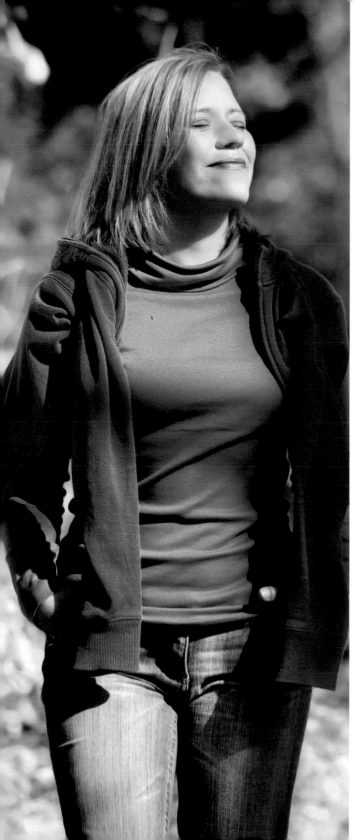

PTH Also Matters

Vitamin D is clearly important for maintaining your weight, but there are other components of sunlight that also influence this. Some of the health problems encountered by a lack of vitamin D can be caused by a hormone called the *parathyroid hormone* (PTH) (124). PTH increases when vitamin D decreases, and it can itself cause insulin resistance and weight gain. PTH even seems to increase blood pressure and the risk of heart disease.

Another consequence of being overweight is that you're less likely to want to show off on the beach, and so you get less exposure to the sun (123). This continues the negative spiral: Reduced levels of vitamin D and increased levels of PTH that in turn cause weight gain.

My Final Sun Tip

Sunshine makes us healthier and helps us burn fat and keep our weight steady. Too much sunshine, though, increases the risk of malignant melanoma and makes the skin age prematurely. My own way of maximizing the benefits of the sun and minimizing damage is to utilize the few hours of sunshine we get during the darker months of the year—fifteen minutes of sunshine to your face on a winter's day actually makes quite a bit of difference

During the summer months or when I am in warmer climes, I never lie in the sun to fry, but prefer to be active out in the sunlight. I make sure to get as much shade as possible, so that I can avoid using sunblock. Sometimes you don't have much choice, and if you're out hiking or at sea and have limited access to shade, you should obviously use sunblock or cover up. Otherwise, it's a good idea to avoid sunblock because it blocks the production of melanocortin. Sunblock is made of quite a few substances that are not great to get into your body; among them are some with undetermined effects on hormones.

If you are the type that really likes to fry in the sun, I'm sure you've weighed the risks against the rewards, and in this case, of course, it's better to use sunblock than to get sunburned or sun poisoning. If you tan, at least you have produced some melanocortin, despite the sunblock.

45

Cut the Stress

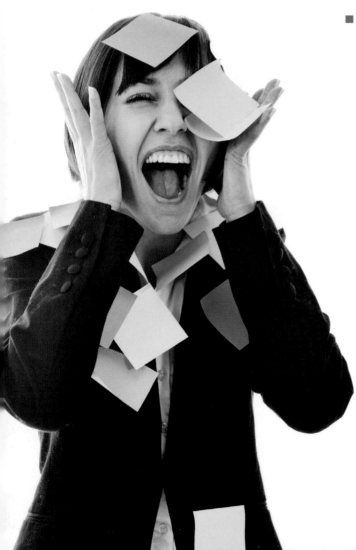

■ A good dose of mental stress keeps us on our toes and makes us perform better. When we feel stressed, adrenaline, norepinephrine, and cortisol are all released, and they quickly release stored energy in the forms of blood sugar and fat to prepare us for fight or flight. This causes an energy spike and temporarily increased alertness and has helped mankind to survive throughout history. The problem is that the stress we encounter today is of a completely different nature and is often much more drawn out and long-term. It might be a matter of being overworked, having financial concerns, or a general feeling of not being "good enough." All of this can cause increased levels of stress hormones, and if they circulate in high amounts over a period of time, the body begins to believe your life is in danger. It interprets the signals as if you've been exposed to long-term danger—something that in the past was related to the risk of dying of starvation. Therefore, over time, stress hormones can cause fat to be stored and sensitivity to insulin to be lowered, allowing the glucose to go to the brain instead of to the muscles. When it comes to a lack of available energy, the brain is considered the most sensitive organ; so when there isn't enough energy to go around, the brain takes priority over the muscles.

Stress Gives You Bad Eating Habits

Whenever there's not enough time in the day, we often become sloppy when it comes to food. We'll eat at irregular times and often won't do so until we're starving.

As you know, when we're famished, we'll grab foods with easily accessed carbohydrates and a lot of fat—chocolates, muffins, hot dogs and fries, hamburgers, etc. We automatically crave calorie-rich foods that are less likely to make us feel full, overlooking homemade food with healthy ingredients. In addition, for many people stress increases appetite, and they will eat to dampen the effects of that stress. This is a form of self-medication that in the long-term will show on the waistline. So, it seems as if people who are stressed need to eat more to feel as full as those who are not stressed.

Stress Makes You Fat

When it comes to long-term stress, cortisol is the main fat building hormone. This is due to the fact that the fat cells absorb more fat when they are exposed to cortisol over the course of weeks and months. A short-term burst of cortisol can actually cause an increased release of fat because it is meant to release energy reserves for temporary strain. But, for long periods of stress, the process flips the other way (248). An increase in cortisol over a longer period of time can also lower insulin sensitivity and, in combination with inactivity, increase the storage of fat in the muscles (247). Intramuscular fat that is forced into your muscles is very unhealthy because it increases the risk of type 2 diabetes. It's a completely different thing when the muscles choose to absorb fat by themselves because that is also related to the increased use of fat as a fuel. When cortisol drives fat into the muscles for extra storage space, this is bad for your health. We also know that cortisol has an especially strong effect on fat storage in the belly, so it's completely possible to stress your way to a paunch (250).

It should, therefore, come as no surprise that research shows a connection between stress and BMI, meaning that stressed people usually weigh more (241, 242, 249).

Some Tips for a Less Stressful Existence

- Practice meditation and do relaxation exercises
- Get moderate exercise
- Make sure you get enough sleep
- Turn off your cell phone and email at certain times during your work day
- Plan ahead for shopping, cooking, etc.

A good book in this subject is *Change Your Thinking: Overcome Stress, Anxiety, and Depression, and Improve Your Life with CBT* by Sarah Edelman.

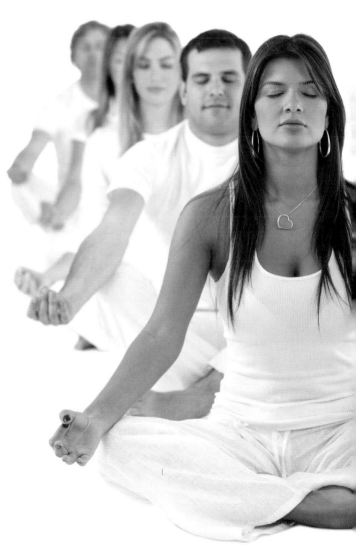

The Two Sides to Nicotine

■ This might seem like a strange shortcut, but I have, in fact, met quite a few people who smoke or use snuff to maintain their weight. Therefore, I think it's an appropriate subject to raise in this book.

There are many opinions surrounding smoking and body weight. Some people claim that smoking keeps them slim, whereas others believe just the opposite. Actually, they're both right! It all depends on the different phases of smoking. If you smoke a cigarette (or take something else containing nicotine), you increase the production of body heat by quite a lot (about a 10-percent higher thermogenesis). So, if your nicotine intake becomes a daily habit, it will eventually keep your weight down. In addition, nicotine releases the neurotransmitter *dopamine* in the brain, which is the same reward-driven substance that rushes in when you do something that creates feelings of pleasure. Sugar, fat, alcohol, sex, shopping, drugs, caffeine, gambling, exercise, and so on, all increase the supply of dopamine to the brain. But, if you get dopamine from nicotine, the need to get it from other sources is reduced. Simply put, smokers will often get full faster.

This becomes evident when people give up smoking. Without tobacco, the focus will shift to food, and this, combined with a lower metabolism, causes weight gain for many people when they give up smoking. However, even a substantial increase in weight is better for your health compared to the long-term effects of smoking (276), so it's definitely a smart decision to give up the habit. As the ideal scenario is to neither get fat nor sick, it's important to get dopamine from other sources, so why not spend more time exercising?

Long-Term Weight Gain from Smoking

Even if nicotine can increase metabolism short-term, smoking is actually a route toward becoming overweight. How does this work? Smoking ultimately means that you ingest so many poisons into your body that you'll slowly but surely lose your sensitivity to insulin. Even nicotine itself seems to lower insulin sensitivity, causing fat to be stored. The more you smoke, the worse the effect. The result is increased weight around the belly and a heightened risk for type 2 diabetes (277). If you want the lovely metabolic syndrome and a paunch to be proud of (including an increased risk of lung cancer), then smoking is a great shortcut (278).

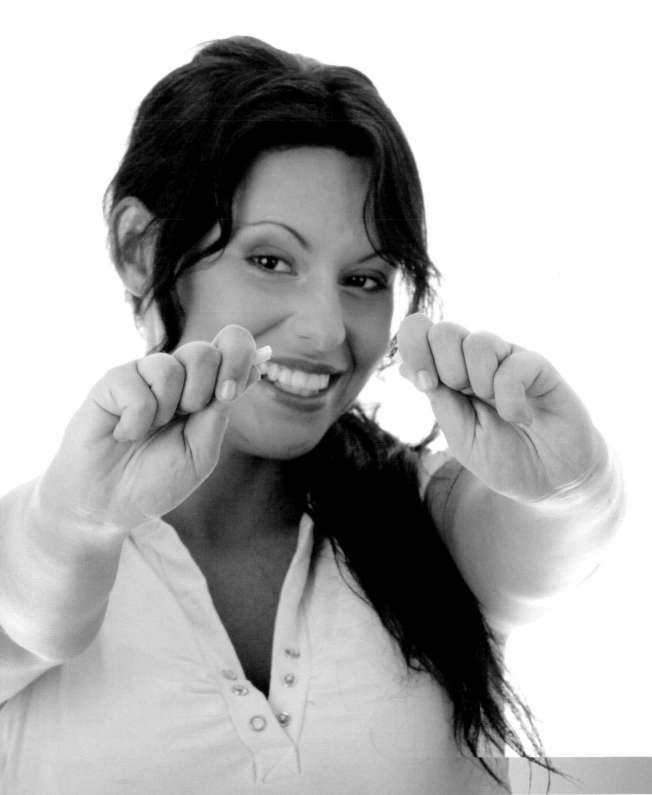

Inhibit Inflammations

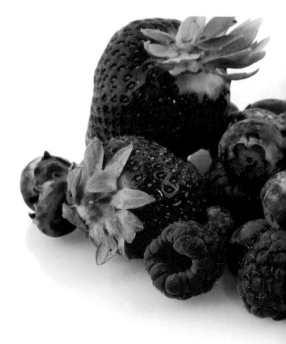

■ Inflammations are vital: When you are hurt, they contract the blood vessels, repair damaged tissue, and produce pain, so that you don't expose an injured body part to more strain. However, too much inflammation isn't good because it increases the risk of heart disease, cancer, dementia, type 2 diabetes, and premature aging.

However, you might be wondering if inflammations can also make you fat. Plenty points to this idea because inflammations reduce insulin sensitivity, which as you know, is crucial when it comes to keeping your weight in balance and burning fat. The fatter we become, the more inflammations we get. And the more inflammations we get, the fatter we become. This is one explanation as to why so many people seem to cross a threshold in their weight gain; once they've passed it, it's hard to go back, and the weight just keeps piling on. This is why it should come as no surprise that many researchers believe a diet that inhibits inflammation will also aid in fat burning and weight loss (292).

Tips to Keep Inflammations at Arm's Length

- Eat in moderation—apart from the risk of excess energy, too many calories release free radicals and activate inflammation. Overweight people who diet will reduce their inflammatory processes (286).

- Eat your greens—as little as 2 lb (1 kg) of vegetables a week gives a measurable anti-inflammatory effect (285). This is due to several factors, such as the presence of salicylates in vegetables. These substances are related to acetylsalicylic acid found in aspirin. In vegetables, however, there are no side effects, and they come in several forms, so the effects are wide-ranging.

- Don't stress out—stress activates your inflammatory processes (287) and is one of the reasons why many become sick from long-term stress.

- Use cold-pressed oil (extra virgin olive oil)—this is packed with nutrients and good fats, but it also contains a high amount of anti-inflammatory substances and is known to be anti-inflamma tory (288).

- Eat at least three portions of oily fish a week—few substances are easier to get that are as effective against inflammations as the omega-3 fats in fish (289).

- Eat magnesium-rich food—it's a mineral that can inhibit inflammation (290). Whole grain products, nuts, coffee, tea, cocoa, spices, and vegetables (especially green, leafy ones) are rich in magnesium.

- Increase your intake of berries—blueberries, blackberries, raspberries, goji berries, blackcurrants, and all other varieties of berries contain natural and powerful anti-inflammatory substances (291). Eat at least 2-4 oz (50-100 g) per day if you can.

- Drink healthy amounts of red wine—as long as you stick to a healthy consumption of red wine, it will have an anti-inflammatory effect. This is partly because of the alcohol itself and partly because of all the antioxidants in wine. Too much, however, will have the opposite effect and will cause you to have more inflammations, so it's important to maintain the balance here.

- Use herbs and spices—many herbs and spices possess powerful anti-inflammatory properties (293). As you have already seen, many herbs and spices also have a direct effect on fat burning and metabolism.

As you can see, there are many similarities between those who wish to lose weight and those who wish to reduce inflammation. It shows how closely these two are linked, and a diet that doesn't try to reduce inflammation will not be as effective at increasing fat burning as a diet that does.

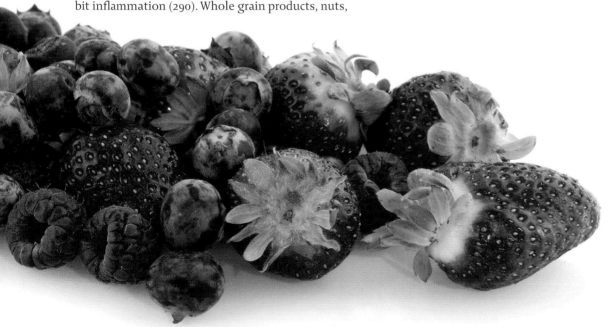

Go Easy on the Sugar

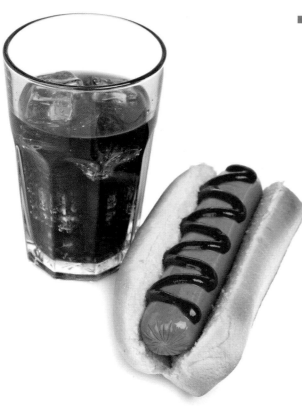

■ I think the most effective shortcut, when you compare the amount of effort required with the result, is to completely exclude plain, white sugar from your food. This is easy to do because sugar ought to always be declared as sugar, glucose, glucose syrup, fructose, syrup, or high fructose corn syrup on the packaging of food. If any of these appear on the label, go with something else.

What happens when you reduce or exclude sugar? Most people who eat sugar regularly have a sugar habit, meaning that their bodies crave sugar every day. This is because of high levels of a hormone known as *ghrelin*. Ghrelin rises after you eat a portion of sugar, and it seems to both stimulate the appetite and increase sugar cravings. If you eat too many sweet things, you'll become used to this; ghrelin will make you drawn to sugar, which will become hard to resist. Because sugar basically means storing fat in its purest form, reducing sugar will quickly give you less body fat. Sugar is very rich in energy, and it has a very high GI value and lacks any form of nutrients (apart from carbohydrates).

There are many different thoughts about how much sugar we really consume on average, but it's not unusual to see figures stating that 20 percent of our energy intake comes from sugar. If you remove this, your

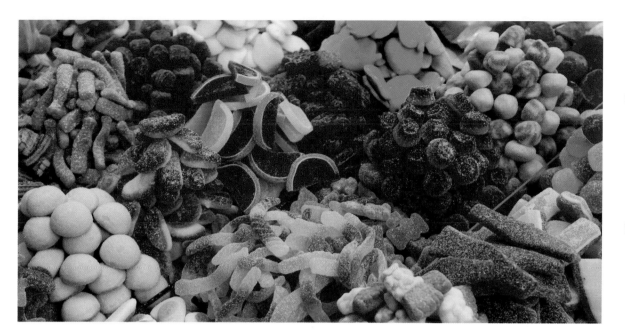

waistline will soon be reduced, even if you eat other things instead. Sugar is the one ingredient that gives the least feeling of fullness per calorie, and you will gain by reducing the amount of sugar you consume. The hardest part of consuming less sugar is the cravings that many will experience, but if you remove sugar and fast-acting carbohydrates, the cravings will subside quite quickly and you'll be on your way to better eating habits.

An Easy Way to Get "Iso-fied"

As you know, I consider it best for health and fitness to eat roughly the same quantity of fats, proteins, and carbohydrates. For most people, this means fewer carbs and more proteins than they are used to. Put simply, becoming "iso-fied."

The easiest way to achieve this, or at least to get on your way, is to skip the sugar and add a bit more protein-rich food. This means you should read all the labels on ready-made foods where sugar might hide: All forms of drinks, bread mixes, cereals, muesli, porridge mixes, cured meats, caviar, soft whey butter, preserves, soy drinks, pasta sauces, powdered products, and dried fruit, to name just a few.

A lot of food found in restaurants contains vast amounts of hidden sugar. Ask at the sushi bar how much sugar there is in the rice, and you'll be surprised at the answer. Thai and Chinese food are often packed with sugar, and even in burger joints you can get too much—especially if you're unaware of the ingredients in the side dishes (and those soda cups aren't exactly small, either).

If you become an avid sugar hunter, it'll be easy to lower your intake, and your ability to burn fat will be more effective. In this case, you can even enjoy some sugar now and again, and you'll really savor your ice cream!

The Scariest of All

Soda is probably the worst thing you can drink if you want to keep a good level of fat burning. Soda contains 9-12 percent carbohydrates in the form of pure sugar, which means that those who drink a 2-liter bottle of soda consume about 240 g of sugar (that's about 20 tablespoons)! Because people often guzzle soda, their blood sugar spikes at an alarming rate. As a result, the strain on glucose levels and the secretion of insulin shoot up to a frightening level, causing an inhibition of fat burning over a longer period.

Because soda does not make you feel full, your energy intake will be much higher when you drink it with your meal than it would be if you had chosen water instead. Not surprisingly, there are a number of studies that show that drinking soda regularly will inhibit fat burning and increase the risk of becoming overweight in both children and adults (251, 252, 255).

The truth is that for many overweight people to start shedding the pounds, drinking less soda is often enough (257). One study showed that 19 percent of the energy intake for overweight people came from high-energy drinks. Nineteen percent is a huge part of your caloric intake! For some reason, when it comes to losing weight, it seems to be more effective to reduce liquid calories than solid ones (257).

Are Sweeteners a Good Alternative?

Many people pick a light alternative when choosing sweets to keep the caloric intake low and the fat burning high. Some have a very liberal point of view when it comes to diet soda and other products sweetened with aspartame, sucralose, acesulfame K, and other synthetic sweeteners. However, it's evident that consuming too much of these will increase the appetite generally—particularly for sweet things (318). Research shows that there is no difference in weight between those who drink diet soda and those who drink regular, sugary soda—and you know how bad full-fat soda is. In my opinion, the only time when light products and sweeteners are okay is when you don't have a choice. Either it's fully-loaded soda (with regular sugar) or diet soda, and in this case, you should choose the latter for your health. Regular soda gives an unnatural amount of blood sugar, which is damaging.

Are sweeteners dangerous? Purely from the perspective of how poisonous they are, sweeteners don't do too much damage and can easily be digested by the body. The exception may be sucralose—due to the chlorine atom, sucralose is harder to digest, and it's still not clear what happens to the body if too much is consumed. We know that it's hard to break down in nature, and it may be a possible threat to the environment. Aspartame is the most researched artificial sweetener and, even if it isn't seen as a health food, it doesn't appear dangerous when consumed in reasonable amounts.

Honey Is a Sin-Free Sweetener

I often have a spoonful of honey in my tea or on my morning porridge if I am craving something sweet. Honey is even perfect in fruit compotes or when roasting your own muesli. The sweet taste is actually very good for you because the brain will flood with reward chemicals such as dopamine, endorphins, and serotonin.

Honey is the complete opposite of white sugar. Despite the actual types of sugars being very similar in these two products, honey gives you much more in the form of antioxidants and trace minerals. One study showed that a daily consumption of 1.2 g honey per kg body weight increased the blood's vitamin C content by 47 percent, beta-carotene by 3 percent, and iron by 20 percent (256). In addition, important antioxidant enzymes increased by 7 percent, and blood sugars sank by 5 percent, whereas zinc and magnesium levels increased significantly.

Sugar actually lowers the levels of nutrients in the body because it increases the consumption of several vitamins and minerals without actually adding anything. Honey also contains the sugar *isomaltulose* (known commercially as palatinose)—an extremely low glycemic source of carbohydrates that has been linked to weight reduction. Palatinose gives a much better rate of fat burning compared to normal sugar (258). Studies of diabetics show that a daily intake of honey over eight weeks actually lowered body weight (259).

Consuming the right type of sugar seems to increase metabolism to the point at which you can lose weight. In addition, you lower your LDL, total cholesterol, and triglycerides in the blood. In another study, subjects had a daily intake of either 2.5 oz (70 g) sugar or of honey over 30 days. The honey group lost 1.3 percent of their weight as well as 1.1 percent body fat. In addition, the LDL, triglycerides, and CRP (a marker for inflammations) were lowered for those who ate honey (260).

How much is good for you depends on your energy expenditure, but use common sense. Personally, I can consume a few tablespoons a day without any problems.

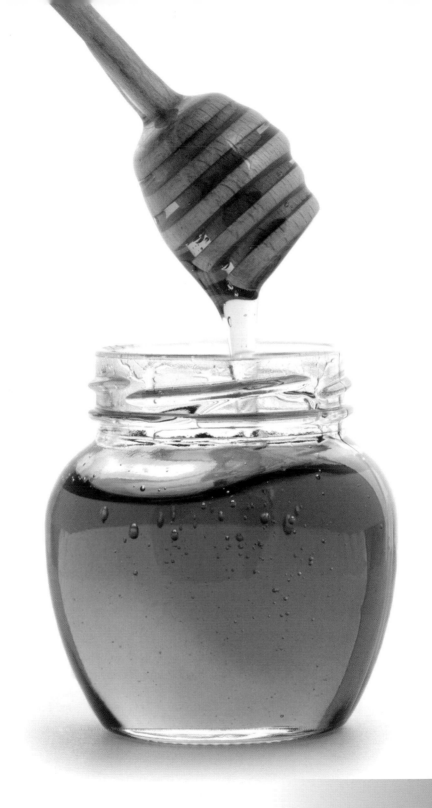

Eat Slowly

There are many reasons why we should eat slowly. One is to reduce our pulse and actually take the time to enjoy our food. Others are to avoid swallowing too much air and to chew everything properly to aid digestion. Those who suffer from bloating after a meal should try to slow down because doing so can help. And perhaps the most compelling reason is that you gain weight when you eat too quickly. Several studies show a positive correlation between the speed at which you eat and weight gain (242, 243, 244, 245, 246).

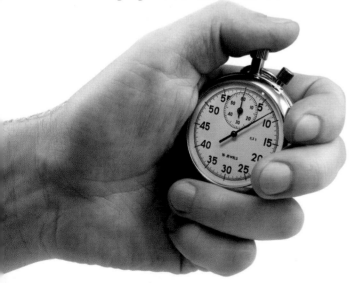

It Takes Fifteen Minutes to Feel Full

It's long been known that it takes a while for the body to register the amount of food consumed. Appetite and the feeling of fullness are very complex systems, which are regulated by both the feeling of fullness in the stomach and that which reaches the blood. Food takes time to digest, and the nutrients take their time reaching the blood. If you stuff yourself full of food in a short period of time, you'll delay the feeling of being full, and you'll have had the time to consume more food than you need. They say it takes fifteen minutes to feel full, and there is much to be said for this statement.

A Faster Increase in Blood Sugar

The more quickly you eat, the faster the food leaves your stomach to be digested in the small intestine. The faster this process takes place, the higher the blood sugar and your insulin levels will rise to keep up. Because high levels of insulin are a risk factor for a lowered insulin sensitivity and type 2 diabetes, it will come as no surprise that people who eat quickly are also affected by a lowered sensitivity to insulin (246). One can also assume that rapid eating is related to stress, and in these cases, you're less likely to make smart choices about food—something that will further affect weight and health.

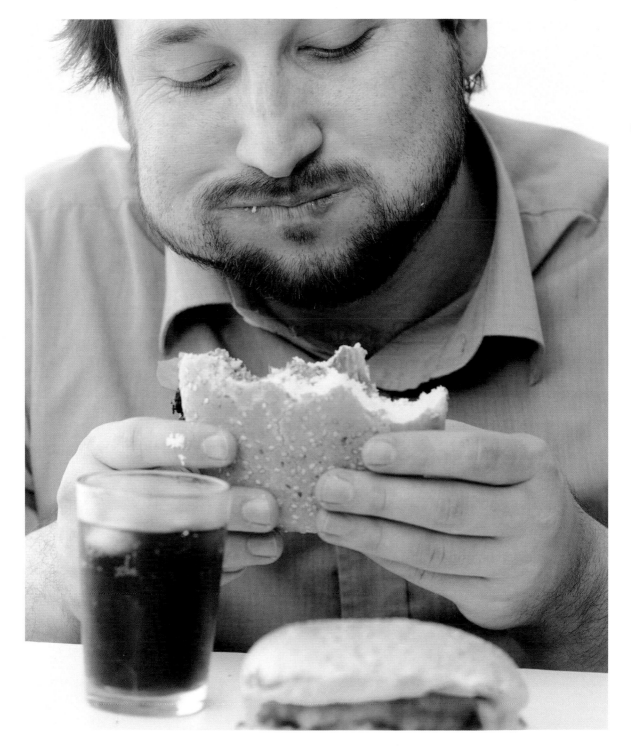

Sleep Your Way into Shape

When I was a studying nutritional physiology, the consensus was that it was beneficial to weight loss to sleep less and have more active hours in the day. Many who wanted to lose weight got out of bed a few hours early and went for walks or exercised. However, it seems that sleep is incredibly important for weight loss and fat burning, and accumulating a sleep debt can actually make you gain weight. Many people who enter into a daily rhythm and get their seven to nine hours of sleep will actually start to lose weight almost spontaneously. Therefore, I think the phrase "sleep your way into shape" is wholly appropriate.

Hunger Increases above Your Expenditure

Many people claim to be hungrier the less sleep they get, and research shows this to be the case. Getting up just a few hours earlier will naturally increase your total energy expenditure over the day because you will be active for more hours. However, your appetite will increase so much that you will eat more calories than you use. Your energy balance becomes what we call *positive*, and you start to gain weight (211). The less sleep you get, the more weight you gain, and after a few months you'll start to notice it around your waistline. The reason for this is that lack of sleep increases the levels of the hormone *ghrelin*, which stimulates your appetite while at the same time reducing *leptin*, a hormone that inhibits appetite. Together, these effects make us feel hungrier.

Several Causes of Hormone Imbalance

Apart from the fact that leptin is reduced and ghrelin increased, even insulin is affected. As you are well aware, insulin is the hormone that regulates blood sugar, and a lack of sleep reduces insulin sensitivity. This results in higher blood sugar levels and an increased risk for type 2 diabetes (212), but also in higher levels of insulin in general. Because insulin is also the hormone that pushes fat into the fat cells, lack of sleep can lead to more effective fat storage—something very few of us want or need. Another consequence is that cortisol levels rise in the evening, and this can stimulate appetite while increasing fat storage at the same time (216). A further hormonal problem is that you release growth hormone during sleep, and this is obviously reduced when sleep is interrupted. As growth hormone has a substantial effect on fat burning, this will slowly lead to weight gain (223). Finally, even glucagon is reduced when there is not enough sleep (236), which effectively lowers your metabolism. Glucagon can be described as the key that unlocks the fat cells, so that fat can enter the muscles and liver to be metabolized.

Moderation Is Best

It's important to keep everything in balance, even when sleeping. Too much sleep isn't good for you either, and those who sleep the longest (more than nine hours a day) also tend to gain weight (213). An extremely long night's sleep might indicate that you're a bit lazy and are less likely to jump out of bed and put on a pair of sneakers. It may also indicate that you're not in full health. An increase in free radicals, which make you tired during infections and inflammations and other states of ill health, can lead to inactivity, lowered metabolism, and an increase in eating. Most adults should get between seven and eight hours sleep per night, with a few needing nine. Very few will benefit from more or less than this.

Research Results

> In one study, twelve men alternated between eight and four hours of sleep per night. The days they only slept four hours, the subjects ate an average of 559 more calories than when they slept for eight hours. In addition, their increased energy expenditure could not reach 559 kcal despite the extra waking hours, so had the study continued, the subjects would likely have increased in weight. The days they slept less, they were also tired the whole day, so even quality of life was negatively affected. (211)

> A Japanese study divided 35, 247 subjects into three groups: those who slept seven to eight hours (the control group) and those who slept either more or less. Those who had the least sleep ran almost twice as much of a risk of becoming overweight as the control. Those who slept the most had about a 50 percent bigger risk than the control, showing that moderation always best (214).

> In one exciting study, subjects were given access to a bed for either 5.5 or 8.5 hours and were given an unlimited amount of food or snacks. Those who had the least sleep tended to eat more calories in the form of snacks compared to those who slept longer (1,087 calories compared with 866 calories, on average). In addition, the lack of sleep increased the consumption of carbohydrates (65 percent compared with 61 percent) (215).

> Even in six-year-old children, lack of sleep can have a negative effect. One Canadian study divided 1,138 six year olds into several groups: those who had fewer than ten consecutive hours of sleep, ten consecutive hours of sleep, and eleven consecutive hours of sleep. Those who got the least sleep had a 4.2 times higher risk of becoming overweight or fat as opposed to those who got eleven consecutive hours sleep (225).

> Even new mothers are affected by sleep. One study showed that women who had fewer than five hours of sleep after giving birth had a difficult time losing weight, and even a year later, they nearly all weighed 11 lb (5 kg) more than before they were pregnant (234).

One of the Most Persuasive Connections

When you examine the science behind various claims, you nearly always find studies that show no effect or even an opposite effect. However, when it comes to looking at the connection between lack of sleep (or even too much sleep) and weight gain, there can be no doubt. This area of research has exploded in the past five years, and about a hundred studies can be found in medical databases that all show (and I have not found anything to the contrary) that you are more likely to get fat if you get too little sleep. Here are some references if you would like some further reading: (215, 217, 218, 219, 220, 221, 226, 227, 228, 229, 230, 231, 232, 233, 235, 237, 238, 239, 240). One interesting question is "Why is it like this?" Why does lack of sleep lead to weight gain? And why are our bodies designed to react in this way? A likely explanation is that it's an evolutionary process. Historically, lack of sleep, just like too much stress, has been linked with hard times, and in these situations, it's good for the body to store fat (222). Hard times often meant starvation, and those who were most able to conserve energy were more likely to survive.

10 Tips for a Better Night's Sleep

1 Keep the room really dark. If possible, use blackout curtains. Placing something over your eyes (a black T-shirt, for example) can also help if you can't get the room dark enough.

2 Keep the room cool. Use different types of duvets depending on the time of year and keep the window wide open to let cool, fresh air in.

3 Make sure it's really quiet. Turn off anything that makes a distracting noise before you go to bed, such as radiators, dripping taps, or electrical equipment.

4 Exercise regularly. Nothing gives you a better night's sleep than exercise. But, don't do so too late at night because you run the risk of being too wound up when it's time to go to bed.

5 Don't drink coffee any later than six hours before bedtime.

6 Adjust your life according to your sleeping pattern as much as possible. There are plenty of examples of how night owls are forced to get up too early and, in this way, accumulate several hours of sleep deprivation each week (a similar problem is being forced to stay up later than your body clock tells you to). Despite this, many people are forced to get up too early. Many times, it is possible to adjust working hours so that they fit our built-in clocks. For some people, it might even be worth choosing a job according to the work hours.

7 Eat something light before you go to bed because this often helps people fall asleep. (See the shortcut on evening eating on page 36).

8 Don't watch television or play on your computer in bed. This will make it harder for the brain to unwind and let you fall asleep.

9 If you are being forced into sleeping less during the week, make sure you compensate for this over the weekend, when you can have a lie-in. Prioritize sleep, so that any deficit causes minimal damage.

10 Make sure your bed is nice and comfortable—after all, you spend a third of your life there! It's worth spending the extra money to get a really good bed.

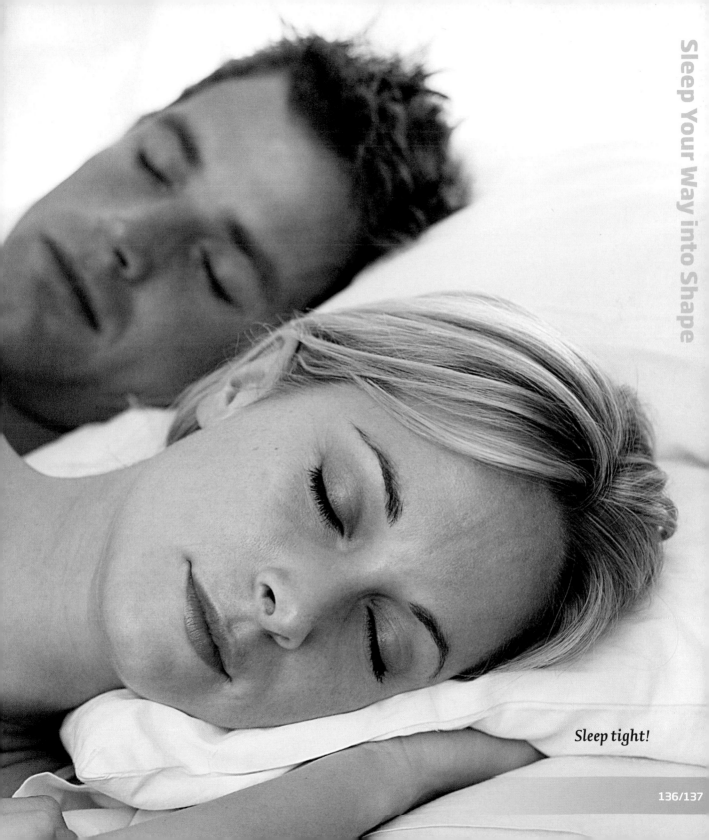

Sleep tight!

References

1 Phung O.J. et al., Effect of green tea catechins with or without caffeine on anthropometric measures: a systematic review and meta-analysis, Am. J. Clin. Nutr. 11, 2009

2 He R.R. et al., Beneficial effects of oolong tea consumption on diet-induced overweight and obese subjects, Chin. J. Integr. Med. 15(1):34-41, 2009

3 Maki K.C. et al., Green tea catechin consumption enhances exercise-induced abdominal fat loss in overweight and obese adults, J. Nutr. 139(2):264-70, 2009

4 Auvichayapat P. et al., Effectiveness of green tea on weight reduction in obese Thais: A randomized, controlled trial, Physiol. Behav. 27;93(3):486-91, 2008

5 Yoshioka M. et al., Effects of red pepper on appetite and energy intake., Br. J. Nutr. 82(2):115-23, 1999

6 Lejeune M.P., Kovacs E.M., Westerterp-Plantenga M.S., Effect of capsaicin on substrate oxidation and weight maintenance after modest body-weight loss in human subjects., Br. J. Nutr. 90(3):651-59, 2003

7 Belza A., Jessen A.B., Bioactive food stimulants of sympathetic activity: effect on 24-h energy expenditure and fat oxidation, Eur. J. Clin. Nutr. 59(6):733-41, 2005

8 Matsumoto T. et al., Effects of capsaicin-containing yellow curry sauce on sympathetic nervous system activity and diet-induced thermogenesis in lean and obese young women., J. Nutr. Sci. Vitaminol 46(6):309-15, 2000

9 Snitker S. et al., Effects of novel capsinoid treatment on fatness and energy metabolism in humans: possible pharmacogenetic implications, Am. J. Clin. Nutr. 89(1):45-50, 2009

10 Yoshioka M. et al., Effects of red pepper added to high-fat and high-carbohydrate meals on energy metabolism and substrate utilization in Japanese women, Br. J. Nutr. 80(6):503-10, 1998

11 Yoshioka M. et al., Effects of red-pepper diet on the energy metabolism in men, J. Nutr. Sci. Vitaminol 41(6):647-56, 1995

12 Hachiya S. et al., Effects of CH-19 Sweet, a non-pungent cultivar of red pepper, on sympathetic nervous activity, body temperature, heart rate, and blood pressure in humans, Biosci. Biotechnol. Biochem. 71(3):671-6, 2007

13 Kawabata F. et al., Effects of CH-19 sweet, a non-pungent cultivar of red pepper, in decreasing the body weight and suppressing body fat accumulation by sympathetic nerve activation in humans, Biosci. Biotechnol. Biochem. 70(12):2824-35, 2006

14 Ahn I.S. et al., Antiobesity effect of Kochujang (Korean fermented red pepper paste) extract in 3T3-L1 adipocytes, J. Med. Food 9(1):15-21, 2006

15 Yoshioka M. et al., Combined effects of red pepper and caffeine consumption on 24 h energy balance in subjects given free access to foods, Br. J. Nutr. 85(2):203-11, 2001

16 Yoshioka M. et al., Effects of red pepper on appetite and energy intake, Br. J. Nutr. 82(2):115-23, 1999

17 Yoshioka M. et al., Effects of red pepper added to high-fat and high-carbohydrate meals on energy metabolism and substrate utilization in Japanese women, Br. J. Nutr. 80(6):503-10, 1998

18 Han L.K. et al., Antiobesity actions of Zingiber officinale Roscoe, Yakugaku Zasshi 125(2):213-7, 2005

19 Westerterp-Plantenga M. et al., Metabolic effects of spices, teas, and caffeine, Physiol Behav. 30;89(1):85-91, 2006

20 Han L.K. et al., Effects of zingerone on fat storage in ovariectomized rats, Yakugaku Zasshi 128(8):1195-201, 2008

21 Henry C.J., Emery B., Effect of spiced food on metabolic rate, Hum. Nutr. Clin. Nutr. 40(2):165-8, 1986

22 Oi Y. et al., Allyl-containing sulfides in garlic increase uncoupling protein content in brown adipose tissue, and noradrenaline and adrenaline secretion in rats, J. Nutr. 129(2):336-42, 1999

23 Elkayam A. et al., The effects of allicin on weight in fructose-induced hyperinsulinemic, hyperlipidemic, hypertensive rats., Am. J. Hypertens 16(12):1053-6, 2003

24 Oi-Kano Y. et al., Oleuropein, a phenolic compound in extra virgin olive oil, increases uncoupling protein 1 content in brown adipose tissue and enhances noradrenaline and adrenaline secretions in rats, J. Nutr. Sci. Vitaminol 54(5):363-70, 2008

25 Jones P.J., Jew S., AbuMweis S., The effect of dietary oleic, linoleic, and linolenic acids on fat oxidation and energy expenditure in healthy men, Metabolism 57(9):1198-203, 2008

26 Piers L.S. et al, The influence of the type of dietary fat on postprandial fat oxidation rates: monounsaturated (olive oil) vs saturated fat (cream), Int. J. Obes. Relat. Metab. Disord. 26(6):814-21, 2002

27 Votruba S.B., Atkinson R.L., Schoeller D.A., Sustained increase in dietary oleic acid oxidation following morning exercise, Int. J. Obes. 29(1):100-7, 2005

28 Bennard P., Doucet E., Acute effects of exercise timing and breakfast meal glycemic index on exercise-induced fat oxidation, Appl. Physiol Nutr. Metab. 31(5):502-11, 2006

29 Bergman B.C., Brooks G.A., Respiratory gas-exchange ratios during graded exercise in fed and fasted trained and untrained men, J. Appl. Physiol. 86(2):479-87, 1999

30 Horswill C. et al., Acute effect of consumption/omission of breakfast on exercise tolerance in adolescents, J. Sports Med. Phys. Fitness 32(1):76-83, 1992

31 Ferguson L.M. et al., Effects of caloric restriction and overnight fasting on cycling endurance performance, J. Strength Cond. Res. 23(2):560-70, 2009

32 Solomon T.P., Blannin A.K., Changes in glucose tolerance and insulin sensitivity following 2 weeks of daily cinnamon ingestion in healthy humans, Eur. J. Appl. Physiol. 105(6):969-76, 2009

33 Ziegenfuss T.N. et al., Effects of a water-soluble cinnamon extract on body composition and features of the metabolic syndrome in pre-diabetic men and women, J. Int. Soc. Sports Nutr. 28;3:45-53, 2006

34 Solomon T.P., Blannin A.K., Effects of short-term cinnamon ingestion on in vivo glucose tolerance, Diabetes Obes. Metab. 9(6):895-901, 2007

35 Hlebowicz J. et al., Effect of cinnamon on postprandial blood glucose, gastric emptying, and satiety in healthy subjects, Am. J. Clin. Nutr. 85(6):1552-6, 2007

36 Wang J.G. et al., The effect of cinnamon extract on insulin resistance parameters in polycystic ovary syndrome: a pilot study, Fertil Steril 88(1):240-3, 2007

37 Mang B. et al., Effects of a cinnamon extract on plasma glucose, HbA, and serum lipids in diabetes mellitus type 2, Eur. J. Clin. Invest. 36(5):340-4, 2006

38 Khan A. et al., Cinnamon improves glucose and lipids of people with type 2 diabetes, Diabetes Care 26(12):3215-8, 2003

39 Westerterp-Plantenga M.S. et al., Dietary protein, weight loss, and weight maintenance, Annu. Rev. Nutr. 29:21-41, 2009

40 Davy B.M. et al., Water consumption reduces energy intake at a breakfast meal in obese older adults, J. Am. Diet Assoc. 108(7):1236-9, 2008

41 Stookey J.D. et al., Drinking water is associated with weight loss in overweight dieting women independent of diet and activity, Obesity 6(11):2481-8, 2008

42 Boschmann M. et al., Water-induced thermogenesis, J. Clin. Endocrinol Metab. 88:6015–6019, 2003

43 Keller U. et al., Effects of changes in hydration on protein, glucose and lipid metabolism in man: impact on health, Eur. J. Clin. Nutr. 57(Suppl 2):S69–74, 2003

44 Bilz S., Ninnis R., Keller U., Effects of hypoosmolality on whole-body lipolysis in man, Metabolism 48:472–476, 1999

45 Hernandez T.L. et al., Lack of suppression of circulating free fatty acids and hypercholesterolemia during weight loss on a high-fat, low-carbohydrate diet, Am. J. Clin. Nutr. 91(3):578-85, 2010

46 Brinkworth G.D. et al., Long-term effects of a very low-carbohydrate diet and a low-fat diet on mood and cognitive function, Arch. Intern Med. 9;169(20):1873-80, 2009

47 White A.M. et al., Blood ketones are directly related to fatigue and perceived effort during exercise in overweight adults adhering to low-carbohydrate diets for weight loss: a pilot study, J. Am. Diet Assoc. 107(10):1792-6, 2007

48 Rosenkranz R.R., Cook C.M., Haub M.D., Endurance training on low-carbohydrate and grain-based diets: a case study, Int. J. Sport Nutr. Exerc. Metab. 17(3):296-309, 2007

49 Qi L. et al., Dietary fibers and glycemic load, obesity, and plasma adiponectin levels in women with type 2 diabetes, Diabetes Care 29(7):1501-5, 2006

50 Mori Y. et al., Role of hypoadiponectinemia in the metabolic syndrome and its association with post-glucose challenge hyper-free fatty acidemia: a study in prediabetic Japanese males, Endocrine 29(2):357-61, 2006

51 Tappy L., Lê K.A., Metabolic effects of fructose and the worldwide increase in obesity, Physiol Rev. 90(1):23-46, 2010

52 Thomas D.E., Elliott E.J., Baur L., Low glycaemic index or low glycaemic load diets for overweight and obesity, Cochrane Database Syst. Rev. 18;(3):CD005105, 2007

53 Szajewska H., Ruszczynski M., Systematic review demonstrating that breakfast consumption influences body weight outcomes in children and adolescents in Europe, Crit. Rev. Food Sci. Nutr. 50(2):113-9, 2010

54 Giovannini M., Agostoni C., Shamir R., Symposium overview: Do we all eat breakfast and is it important? Crit. Rev. Food Sci. Nutr. 50(2):97-9, 2010

55 Scazzina F. The effect of breakfasts varying in glycemic index and glycemic load on dietary induced thermogenesis and respiratory quotient, Nutr. Metab. Cardiovasc. Dis. 14, 2009

56 MacFarlane A. et al., Longitudinal examination of the family food environment and weight status among children, Int. J. Pediatr. Obes. 4(4):343-52, 2009

57 Gordon M.M. et al., Effects of dietary protein on the composition of weight loss in post-menopausal women, J. Nutr. Health Aging 12(8):505-9, 2008

58 Sen B., Frequency of family dinner and adolescent body weight status: evidence from the national longitudinal survey of youth, 1997, Obesity 14(12):2266-76, 2006

59 Hsu T.F. et al., Polyphenol-enriched oolong tea increases fecal lipid excretion, Eur. J. Clin. Nutr. 60(11):1330-6, 2006

60 Greenberg J.A., Boozer C.N., Geliebter A., Coffee, diabetes, and weight control, Am. J. Clin. Nutr. 84(4):682-93, 2006

61 Petrie H.J. et al., Caffeine ingestion increases the insulin response to an oral-glucose-tolerance test in obese men before and after weight loss, Am. J. Clin. Nutr. 80(1):22-8, 2004

62 Zhang Y. et al., Coffee consumption and the incidence of type 2 diabetes in men and women with normal glucose tolerance: The Strong Heart Study, Nutr. Metab. Cardiovasc. Dis. 17, 2010

63 Huxley R. et al., Coffee, decaffeinated coffee, and tea consumption in relation to incident type 2 diabetes mellitus: A systematic review with meta-analysis, Arch. Intern Med. 14;169(22):2053-63, 2009

64 Acheson K.J. et al., Metabolic effects of caffeine in humans: lipid oxidation or futile cycling? Am. J. Clin. Nutr. 79(1):40-6, 2004

65 van Dijk A.E. et al., Acute effects of decaffeinated coffee and the major coffee components chlorogenic acid and trigonelline on glucose tolerance, Diabetes Care 32(6):1023-5, 2009

66 Kwon do Y. et al., Comparison of peroxyl radical scavenging capacity of commonly consumed beverages, Arch. Pharm. Res. 32(2):283-7, 2009

67 Thom E., The effect of chlorogenic acid enriched coffee on glucose absorption in healthy volunteers and its effect on body mass when used long-term in overweight and obese people, J. Int. Med. Res. 35(6):900-8, 2007

68 Dallas C. et al., Lipolytic effect of a polyphenolic citrus dry extract of red orange, grapefruit, orange (SINETROL) in human body fat adipocytes. Mechanism of action by inhibition of cAMP-phosphodiesterase (PDE), Phytomedicine 15(10):783-92, 2008

69 Fujioka K. et al., The effects of grapefruit on weight and insulin resistance: relationship to the metabolic syndrome, J. Med. Food 9(1):49-54, 2006

70 Shen J. et al., Olfactory stimulation with scent of grapefruit oil affects autonomic nerves, lipolysis and appetite in rats, Neurosci Lett. 3;380(3):289-94, 2005

71 Niijima A., Nagai K., Effect of olfactory stimulation with flavor of grapefruit oil and lemon oil on the activity of sympathetic branch in the white adipose tissue of the epididymis, Exp. Biol. Med. 228(10):1190-2, 2003

72 Rodríguez-Rodríguez E. et al., Associations between abdominal fat and body mass index on vitamin D status in a group of Spanish schoolchildren, Eur. J. Clin. Nutr. 10, 2010

73 Sergeev I.N., 1,25-Dihydroxyvitamin D3 induces Ca2+-mediated apoptosis in adipocytes via activation of calpain and caspase-12, Biochem Biophys. Res. Commun. 19;384(1):18-21, 2009

74 Major G.C. et al., Calcium plus vitamin D supplementation and fat mass loss in female very low calcium consumers: potential link with a calcium specific appetite control, Br. J. Nutr. 101(5):659-63, 2009

75 Sneve M., Figenschau Y., Jorde R., Supplementation with cholecalciferol does not result in weight reduction in overweight and obese subjects, Eur. J. Endocrinol. 159(6):675-84, 2008

76 Teegarden D. et al., Calcium and dairy product modulation of lipid utilization and energy expenditure, Obesity 16(7):1566-72, 2008

77 Gilsanz V. et al., Vitamin D Status and Its Relation to Muscle Mass and Muscle Fat in Young Women, J. Clin. Endocrinol Metab. 17, 2010

78 Annweiler C. et al., Vitamin D-related changes in physical performance: a systematic review, J. Nutr. Health Aging 13(10):893-8, 2009

79 Hargrave K.M., Azain M.J., Miner J.L., Dietary coconut oil increases conjugated linoleic acid-induced body fat loss in mice independent of essential fatty acid deficiency, Biochim. Biophys. Acta 15;1737(1):52-60, 2005

80 Assunção M.L. etal., Effects of dietary coconut oil on the biochemical and anthropometric profiles of women presenting abdominal obesity, Lipids 44(7):593-601, 2009

81 Papamandjaris A.A., Endogenous fat oxidation during medium chain versus long chain triglyceride feeding in healthy women, Int. J. Obes. Relat. Metab. Disord. 24(9):1158-66, 2000

82 Portillo M.P. et al., Energy restriction with high-fat diet enriched with coconut oil gives higher UCP1 and lower white fat in rats, Int. J. Obes. Relat. Metab. Disord. 22(10):974-9, 1998

83 St-Onge M.P., Bosarge A., Weight-loss diet that includes consumption of medium-chain triacylglycerol oil leads to a greater rate of weight and fat mass loss than does olive oil, Am. J. Clin. Nutr. 87(3):621-6, 2008

84 Han J.R. et al., Effects of dietary medium-chain triglyceride on weight loss and insulin sensitivity in a group of moderately overweight free-living type 2 diabetic Chinese subjects, Metabolism 56(7):985-91, 2007

85 St-Onge M.P., Jones P.J., Greater rise in fat oxidation with medium-chain triglyceride consumption relative to long-chain triglyceride is associated with lower initial body weight and greater loss of subcutaneous adipose tissue, Int. J. Obes. Relat. Metab. Disord. 27(12):1565-71, 2003

86 St-Onge M.P. et al., Medium-chain triglycerides increase energy expenditure and decrease adiposity in overweight men, Obes. Res. 11(3):395-402, 2003

87 St-Onge M.P. et al., Medium- versus long-chain triglycerides for 27 days increases fat oxidation and energy expenditure without resulting in changes in body composition in overweight women. Int. J. Obes. Relat. Metab. Disord. 27(1):95-102, 2003

88 Tsuji H. et al., Dietary medium-chain triacylglycerols suppress accumulation of body fat in a double-blind, controlled trial in healthy men and women, J. Nutr. 131(11):2853-9, 2001

89 Faghih S. et al., Comparison of the effects of cows' milk, fortified soy milk, and calcium supplement on weight and fat loss in premenopausal overweight and obese women, Nutr. Metab. Cardiovasc. Dis. 11, 2010

90 Bush N.C. et al., Dietary Calcium Intake Is Associated With Less Gain in Intra-Abdominal Adipose Tissue Over 1 Year, Obesity 4, 2010

91 Major G.C. et al., Calcium plus vitamin D supplementation and fat mass loss in female very low-calcium consumers: potential link with a calcium-specific appetite control, Br. J. Nutr. 101(5):659-63, 2009

92 Demling R.H., DeSanti L., Effect of a hypocaloric diet, increased protein intake and resistance training on lean mass gains and fat mass loss in overweight police officers, Ann. Nutr. Metab. 44(1):21-9, 2009

93 Claessens M. et al., The effect of a low-fat, high-protein or high-carbohydrate ad libitum diet on weight loss maintenance and metabolic risk factors, Int. J. Obes. 33(3):296-304, 2009

94 Cribb P.J. et al., The effect of whey isolate and resistance training on strength, body composition, and plasma glutamine, Int. J. Sport Nutr. Exerc. Metab. 16(5):494-509, 2006

95 Van Loan M., The role of dairy foods and dietary calcium in weight management, J. Am. Coll. Nutr. 28 Suppl 1:120S-9S, 2006

96 Christensen R. et al., Effect of calcium from dairy and dietary supplements on faecal fat excretion: a meta-analysis of randomized controlled trials, Obes. Rev. 10(4):475-86, 2009

97 Lanou A.J, Barnard N.D., Dairy and weight loss hypothesis: an evaluation of the clinical trials, Nutr. Rev. 66(5):272-9, 2008

98 de Castro J.M., The time of day of food intake influences overall intake in humans, J. Nutr. 134(1):104-11, 2004

99 Calugi S., Dalle Grave R., Marchesini G., Night eating syndrome in class II-III obesity: metabolic and psychopathological features, Int. J. Obes. 33(8):899-904, 2009

100 Andersen G.S. et al., Night eating and weight change in middle-aged men and women, Int. J. Obes. Relat. Metab. Disord. 28(10):1338-43, 2004

101 Gluck M.E., Geliebter A., Satov T., Night eating syndrome is associated with depression, low self-esteem, reduced daytime hunger, and less weight loss in obese outpatients, Obes. Res. 9(4):264-7, 2001

102 Cope M.B. et al., The potential role of soyfoods in weight and adiposity reduction: an evidence-based review, Obes. Rev. 9(3):219-35, 2008

103 Xiao C. et al., Differential effects of monounsaturated, polyunsaturated and saturated fat ingestion on glucose-stimulated insulin secretion, sensitivity and clearance in overweight and obese, non-diabetic humans, Diabetologia 49(6):1371–1379, 2006

104 Robertson M.D. et al., Acute effects of meal fatty acid composition on insulin sensitivity in healthy post-menopausal women, Br. J. Nutr. 88(6):635–640, 2002

105 Mamalakis G. et al., Abdominal vs buttock adipose fat: relationships with children's serum lipid levels, Eur. J. Clin. Nutr. 56(11):1081–1086, 2002

106 Votruba S.B., Atkinson R.L., Schoeller D.A., Prior exercise increases dietary oleate, but not palmitate oxidation, Obes. Res. 11(12):1509–1518, 2003

107 Xiao C. et al., Differential effects of monounsaturated, polyunsaturated and saturated fat ingestion on glucose-stimulated insulin secretion, sensitivity and clearance in overweight and obese, non-diabetic humans, Diabetologia 49(6):1371–1379, 2006

108 Piers L.S. et al., Substitution of saturated with monounsaturated fat in a 4-week diet affects body weight and composition of overweight and obese men, Br. J. Nutr. 90(3):717–727, 2003

109 Mitchell D. et al., Body composition in the elderly: the influence of nutritional factors and physical activity, J. Nutr. Health Aging 7(3):130–139, 2003

110 Casas-Agustench P. et al., Acute effects of three high-fat meals with different fat saturations on energy expenditure, substrate oxidation and satiety, Clin. Nutr. 28(1):39-45, 2009

111 Ogawa A. et al., Dietary medium- and long-chain triacylglycerols accelerate diet-induced thermogenesis in humans, J. Oleo Sci. 56(6):283-7, 2007

112 van Marken Lichtenbelt W.D., Mensink R.P., Westerterp K.R., The effect of fat composition of the diet on energy metabolism, Z. Ernahrungswiss. 36(4):303-5, 1997

113 Tappy L., Thermic effect of food and sympathetic nervous system activity in humans, Reprod. Nutr. Dev. 36(4):391-7, 1996

114 Jones P.J., Schoeller D.A., Polyunsaturated: saturated ratio of diet fat influences energy substrate utilization in the human, Metabolism 37(2):145-51, 1988

115 Labayen I. et al., Basal and postprandial substrate oxidation rates in obese women receiving two test meals with different protein content, Clin. Nutr. 23(4):571-8, 1988

116 Fernández de la Puebla R.A. et al., A reduction in dietary saturated fat decreases body fat content in overweight, hypercholesterolemic males, Nutr. Metab. Cardiovasc. Dis. 13(5):273-7, 2003

117 Summers L.K. et al., Substituting dietary saturated fat with polyunsaturated fat changes abdominal fat distribution and improves insulin sensitivity, Diabetologia 45(3):369-77, 2002

118 Soares M.J. et al., The acute effects of olive oil v. cream on postprandial thermogenesis and substrate oxidation in postmenopausal women, Br. J. Nutr. 91(2):245-52, 2004

119 Romon M. et al., Circadian variation of diet-induced thermogenesis, Am. J. Clin. Nutr. 57(4):476-80, 1993

120 McGill A.T. et al., Relationships of low serum vitamin D3 with anthropometry and markers of the metabolic syndrome and diabetes in overweight and obesity, Nutr. J. 28;7:4, 2008

121 Moschonis G. et al., Association between serum 25-hydroxyvitamin D levels and body composition in postmenopausal women: the postmenopausal Health Study, Menopause 16(4):701-7, 2009

122 McKinney K., Breitkopf C.R., Berenson A.B., Association of race, body fat and season with vitamin D status among young women: a cross-sectional study, Clin. Endocrinol. 69(4):535-41, 2008

123 Kull M., Kallikorm R., Lember M., Body mass index determines sunbathing habits: implications on vitamin D levels, Intern. Med. J. 39(4):256-8, 2009

124 McCarty M.F., Thomas C.A., PTH excess may promote weight gain by impeding catecholamine-induced lipolysis-implications for the impact of calcium, vitamin D, and alcohol on body weight, Med. Hypotheses. 61(5-6):535-42, 2003

125 Wang L. et al., Alcohol consumption, weight gain, and risk of becoming overweight in middle-aged and older women, Arch. Intern. Med. 8;170(5):453-61, 2010

126 Yeomans M.R., Alcohol, appetite and energy balance: Is alcohol intake a risk factor for obesity? Physiol. Behav. 22, 2010

127 Sieri S. et al., Alcohol consumption patterns, diet and body weight in 10 European countries, Eur. J. Clin. Nutr. 63 Suppl 4:S81-100, 2009

128 Beulens J.W., Effect of moderate alcohol consumption on adipokines and insulin sensitivity in lean and overweight men: a diet intervention study, Eur. J. Clin. Nutr. 62(9):1098-105, 2008

129 Beulens J.W. et al., The effect of moderate alcohol consumption on adiponectin oligomers and muscle oxidative capacity: a human intervention study, Diabetologia 50(7):1388-92, 2007

130 Arif A.A., Rohrer J.E., Patterns of alcohol drinking and its association with obesity: data from the Third National Health and Nutrition Examination Survey, 1988–1994, BMC Public Health 5;5:126, 2005

131 Suter P.M., Is alcohol consumption a risk factor for weight gain and obesity? Crit. Rev. Clin. Lab. Sci. 42(3):197-227, 2005

132 Flechtner-Mors M. et al., Effects of moderate consumption of white wine on weight loss in overweight and obese subjects, Int. J. Obes. Relat. Metab. Disord. 28(11):1420-6, 2004

133 Sierksma A. et al., Effect of moderate alcohol consumption on adiponectin, tumor necrosis factor-alpha, and insulin sensitivity, Diabetes Care 27(1):184-9, 2004

134 Wannamethee S.G. et al., Alcohol consumption and the incidence of type II diabetes. J. Epidemiol. Community Health 56(7):542-8, 2002

135 Davies M.J. et al., Effects of moderate alcohol intake on fasting insulin and glucose concentrations and insulin sensitivity in postmenopausal women: a randomized controlled trial, JAMA 15;287(19):2559-62, 2002

136 Imhof A. et al., Effect of drinking on adiponectin in healthy men and women: a randomized intervention study of water, ethanol, red wine, and beer with or without alcohol, Diabetes Care 32(4):1101-3, 2009

137 Ramel A. et al., Beneficial effects of long-chain n-3 fatty acids included in an energy-restricted diet on insulin resistance in overweight and obese European young adults, Diabetologia 51(7):1261-8, 2008

138 Ramel A., Jonsdottir M.T., Thorsdottir I., Consumption of cod and weight loss in young overweight and obese adults on an energy reduced diet for 8-weeks, Nutr. Metab. Cardiovasc. Dis. 19(10):690-6, 2009

139 Thorsdottir I. Et al., Randomized trial of weight-loss-diets for young adults varying in fish and fish oil content, Int. J. Obes. 31(10):1560-6, 2007

140 Abete I., Parra D., Martinez J.A., Legume-, fish-, or high-protein-based hypocaloric diets: effects on weight loss and mitochondrial oxidation in obese men, J. Med. Food 12(1):100-8, 2009

141 Cassady B.A. et al., Effects of low carbohydrate diets high in red meats or poultry, fish and shellfish on plasma lipids and weight loss, Nutr. Metab. 31;4:23, 2007

142 Parra D. et al., A diet rich in long chain omega-3 fatty acids modulates satiety in overweight and obese volunteers during weight loss, Appetite 51(3):676-80, 2008

143 Ratliff J. et al., Consuming eggs for breakfast influences plasma glucose and ghrelin, while reducing energy intake during the next 24 hours in adult men, Nutr. Res. 30(2):96-103, 2010

144 Vander Wal J.S. et al., Short-term effect of eggs on satiety in overweight and obese subjects, J. Am. Coll. Nutr. 24(6):510-5, 2005

145 Mattes R.D., Dreher M.L., Nuts and healthy body weight maintenance mechanisms, Asia Pac. J. Clin. Nutr. (1):137-41, 2010

146 Casas-Agustench P., Bullo M., Salas-Salvado J., Nuts, inflammation and insulin resistance, Asia Pac. J. Clin. Nutr. 19(1):124-30, 2010

147 Sabaté J., Ang Y., Nuts and health outcomes: new epidemiologic evidence, Am. J. Clin. Nutr. 89(5):1643S-1648S, 2009

148 Natoli S., McCoy P., A review of the evidence: nuts and body weight, Asia Pac. J. Clin. Nutr. 16(4):588-97, 2007

149 Casas-Agustench P. et al., Effects of one serving of mixed nuts on serum lipids, insulin resistance and inflammatory markers in patients with the metabolic syndrome, Nutr. Metab. Cardiovasc. Dis. 21, 2009

150 Bes-Rastrollo M. et al., Prospective study of nut consumption, long-term weight change, and obesity risk in women, Am. J. Clin. Nutr. 89(6):1913-9, 2009

151 Cassady B.A. et al., Mastication of almonds: effects of lipid bioaccessibility, appetite, and hormone response, Am. J. Clin. Nutr. 89(3):794-800, 2009

152 Mattes R.D., Kris-Etherton P.M., Foster G.D., Impact of peanuts and tree nuts on body weight and healthy weight loss in adults, J. Nutr. 138(9):1741S-1745S, 2008

153 Mattes R.D., The energetics of nut consumption, Asia Pac. J. Clin. Nutr. Suppl 1:337-9, 2008

154 Bes-Rastrollo M. et al., Nut consumption and weight gain in a Mediterranean cohort: The SUN study, Obesity 15(1):107-16, 2008

155 Rajaram S., Sabaté J., Nuts, body weight and insulin resistance, Br. J. Nutr. 96 Suppl 2:S79-86, 2006

156 Sabaté J., Nut consumption and body weight, Am. J. Clin. Nutr. 78(3 Suppl):647S-650S, 2003

157 Hollis J., Mattes R., Effect of chronic consumption of almonds on body weight in healthy humans, Br. J. Nutr. 98(3):651-6, 2007

158 Jenkins D.J. et al., Effect of almonds on insulin secretion and insulin resistance in nondiabetic hyperlipidemic subjects: a randomized controlled crossover trial, Metabolism 57(7):882-7, 2008

159 Wien M.A. et al., Almonds vs complex carbohydrates in a weight reduction program, Int. J. Obes. Relat. Metab. Disord. 27(11):1365-72, 2003

160 Sabaté J. et al., Does regular walnut consumption lead to weight gain? Br. J. Nutr. 94(5):859-64, 2005

161 Claesson A.L. et al., Two weeks of overfeeding with candy, but not peanuts, increases insulin levels and body weight, Scand. J. Clin. Lab. Invest. 69(5):598-605, 2009

162 Hill J.O. et al., Obesity and the environment: where do we go from here? Science 299:853-855, 2003

163 Field A.E. et al., Dietary fat and weight gain among women in the Nurse´s Health Study, Obesity 15:967-976, 2007

164 Newby P.K. et al., Intake of whole grains, refined grains, and cereal fiber measured with 7-d diet records and association with risk factors for chronic disease, Am. J. Clin. Nutr. 86:1745-1753, 2007

165 Lutsey P.L. et al., Whole grain intake and its cross-sectional association with obesity, insulin resistance, inflammation, diabetes and subclinical CVD: The MESA Study, Br. J. Nutr. 98:397-405, 2007

166 Good C.K. et al., Whole grain consumption and body mass index in adult women: an analysis of NHANES 1999-2000 and the USDA Pyramid Servings Database, J. Am. Coll. Nutr. 27:80-87, 2008

167 McKeown N.M. et al., Whole-grain intake is favorably associated with metabolic risk factors for type 2 diabetes and cardiovascular disease in the Framingham Offspring Study, Am. J. Clin. Nutr. 76:390-398, 2002

168 Sahyoun N.R. et al., Whole-grain intake is inversely associated with the metabolic syndrome and mortality in older adults, Am. J. Clin. Nutr. 83: 124-131, 2006

169 Murakami K. et al., Dietary fiber intake, dietary glycemic index and load, and body mass index: a cross-sectional study of 3931 Japanese women aged 18–20 years, Eur. J. Clin. Nutr. 61:986-995, 2007

170 Liese A.D. et al., Dietary glycemic index and glycemic load, carbohydrate and fiber intake, and measures of insulin sensitivity, secretion, and adiposity in the Insulin Resistance Atherosclerosis Study, Diabetes Care 28: 2832-2838, 2005

171 Norris L.E. et al., Comparison of dietary conjugated linoleic acid with safflower oil on body composition in obese postmenopausal women with type 2 diabetes mellitus, Am. J. Clin. Nutr. 90(3):468-76, 2009

172 Rahman M., Conjugated linoleic acid (CLA) prevents age-associated skeletal muscle loss, Biochem. Biophys. Res. Commun. 12;383(4):513-8, 2009

173 Li J.J., Huang C.J., Xie D., Anti-obesity effects of conjugated linoleic acid, docosahexaenoic acid, and eicosapentaenoic acid, Mol. Nutr. Food Res. 52(6):631-45, 2008

174 Thrush A.B. et al., Conjugated linoleic acid increases skeletal muscle ceramide content and decreases insulin sensitivity in overweight, non-diabetic humans, Appl. Physiol. Nutr. Metab. 32(3):372-82, 2007

175 Whigham L.D., Watras A.C., Schoeller D.A., Efficacy of conjugated linoleic acid for reducing fat mass: a meta-analysis in humans, Am. J. Clin. Nutr. 85(5):1203-11, 2007

176 Gaullier J.M. et al., Six months supplementation with conjugated linoleic acid induces regional-specific fat mass decreases in overweight and obese, Br. J. Nutr. 97(3):550-60, 2007

177 Gaullier J.M. et al., Supplementation with conjugated linoleic acid for 24 months is well tolerated by and reduces body fat mass in healthy, overweight humans, J. Nutr. 135(4):778-84, 2005

178 Risérus U. et al., Effects of cis-9, trans-11 conjugated linoleic acid supplementation on insulin sensitivity, lipid peroxidation, and proinflammatory markers in obese men, Am. J. Clin. Nutr. 80(2):279-83, 2004

179 Kamphuis M.M. et al., Effect of conjugated linoleic acid supplementation after weight loss on appetite and food intake in overweight subjects, Eur. J. Clin. Nutr. 57(10):1268-74, 2003

180 Kamphuis M.M. et al., The effect of conjugated linoleic acid supplementation after weight loss on body weight regain, body composition, and resting metabolic rate in overweight subjects, Int. J. Obes. Relat. Metab. Disord. 27(7):840-7, 2003

181 Kennedy A. et al., Antiobesity mechanisms of action of conjugated linoleic acid, J. Nutr. Biochem. 21(3):171-9, 2010

182 Steck S.E. et al., Conjugated linoleic acid supplementation for twelve weeks increases lean body mass in obese humans, J. Nutr. 137(5):1188-93, 2007

183 Syvertsen C. et al., The effect of 6 months supplementation with conjugated linoleic acid on insulin resistance in overweight and obese, Int. J. Obes. 31(7):1148-54, 2007

184 Desroches S. et al., Lack of effect of dietary conjugated linoleic acids naturally incorporated into butter on the lipid profile and body composition of overweight and obese men, Am. J. Clin. Nutr. 82(2):309-19, 2005

185 Whigham L.D. et al., Safety profile of conjugated linoleic acid in a 12-month trial in obese humans, Food Chem. Toxicol. 42(10):1701-9, 2004

186 Chevassus H. et al., A fenugreek seed extract selectively reduces spontaneous fat consumption in healthy volunteers, Eur. J. Clin. Pharmacol. 65(12):1175-8, 2009

187 Sharma R.D., Raghuram T.C., Rao N.S., Effect of fenugreek seeds on blood glucose and serum lipids in type I diabetes, Eur. J. Clin. Nutr. 44(4):301-6, 1990

188 Losso J.N. et al., Fenugreek bread: a treatment for diabetes mellitus, J. Med. Food 12(5):1046-9, 2009

189 Wycherley T.P. et al., A high protein diet with resistance exercise training improves weight loss and body composition in overweight and obese patients with type 2 diabetes, Diabetes Care 11, 2010

190 Kerksick C. et al., Effects of a popular exercise and weight loss program on weight loss, body composition, energy expenditure and health in obese women, Nutr. Metab. 14;6:23, 2009

191 Nygaard H., Tomten S.E., Høstmark A.T., Slow postmeal walking reduces postprandial glycemia in middle-aged women, Appl. Physiol. Nutr. Metab. 34(6):1087-92, 2009

192 O'Neil C.E., Nicklas T.A., Kleinman R., Relationship between 100 % juice consumption and nutrient intake and weight of adolescents, Am. J. Health Promot. 24(4):231-7, 2010

193 Schroder K.E., Effects of fruit consumption on body mass index and weight loss in a sample of overweight and obese dieters enrolled in a weight-loss intervention trial, Nutrition 17, 2009

194 Sartorelli D.S., Franco L.J., Cardoso M.A., High intake of fruits and vegetables predicts weight loss in Brazilian overweight adults, Nutr. Res. 28(4):233-8, 2008

195 Vioque J. et al., Intake of fruits and vegetables in relation to 10-year weight gain among Spanish adults, Obesity 16(3):664-70, 2008

196 Bes-Rastrollo M. Et al., Association of fiber intake and fruit/vegetable consumption with weight gain in a Mediterranean population, Nutrition 22(5):504-11, 2006

197 He K. et al., Changes in intake of fruits and vegetables in relation to risk of obesity and weight gain among middle-aged women, Int. J. Obes. Relat. Metab. Disord. 28(12):1569-74, 2004

198 Alinia S., Hels O., Tetens I., The potential association between fruit intake and body weight – a review, Obes. Rev. 10(6):639-47, 2009

199 Shenoy S.F. e.al., Weight loss in individuals with metabolic syndrome given DASH diet counseling when provided a low sodium vegetable juice: a randomized controlled trial, Nutr. J. 23;9:8, 2010

200 Wycherley T.P. et al., A high protein diet with resistance exercise training improves weight loss and body composition in overweight and obese patients with type 2 diabetes, Diabetes Care 11, 2010

201 Acheson K.J., Carbohydrate for weight and metabolic control: where do we stand? Nutrition 26(2):141-5, 2010

202 Henry C.J., Piggot S.M., Effect of ginger on metabolic rate, Hum. Nutr. Clin. Nutr. 41;89-92, 1987

203 Macarulla M.T. et al., Effects of different doses of resveratrol on body fat and serum parameters in rats fed a hypercaloric diet, J. Physiol. Biochem. 65(4):369-76, 2009

204 McKiernan F. et al., Effects of peanut processing on body weight and fasting plasma lipids, Br. J. Nutr. 11:1-9, 2010

205 Clarke S.D. et al., Polyunsaturated fatty acid inhibition of fatty acid synthase transcription is independent of PPAR activation, Z. Ernahrungswiss. 37, Suppl. 1: 14-20, 1998

206 Conner W.E. et al., Differential mobilization of fatty acids from adipose tissue, J. Lipid Res. 37(2):290-8, 1996

207 Forsythe W.A., Soy protein, thyroid regulation and cholesterol metabolism, J. Nutr. 125, (3 suppl): 619-623, 1995

208 Liu Z.M. et al., A mild favorable effect of soy protein with isoflavones on body composition – a 6-month double-blind randomized placebo-controlled trial among Chinese postmenopausal women, Int. J. Obes. 34(2):309-18, 2010

209 Maskarinec G. Et al., Soy intake is related to a lower body mass index in adult women, Eur. J. Nutr. 47(3):138-44, 2008

210 Cope M.B., Erdman J.W. Jr, Allison D.B., The potential role of soyfoods in weight and adiposity reduction: an evidence-based review, Obes. Rev. 9(3):219-35, 2008

211 Brondel L. et al., Acute partial sleep deprivation increases food intake in healthy men, Am. J. Clin. Nutr. 91(6):1550-9, 2010

212 Knutson K.L., Van Cauter E., Associations between sleep loss and increased risk of obesity and diabetes, Ann. N Y Acad. Sci. 1129:287-304, 2008

213 Hairston K.G. et al., Sleep duration and five-year abdominal fat accumulation in a minority cohort: the IRAS family study, Sleep 1;33(3):289-95, 2010

214 Watanabe M. et al., Association of short sleep duration with weight gain and obesity at 1-year follow-up: a large-scale prospective study, Sleep 1;33(2):161-7, 2010

215 Shaikh W.A., Patel M., Singh S., Sleep deprivation predisposes gujarati Indian adolescents to obesity, Indian J. Community Med. 34(3):192-4, 2009

216 Leproult R., Van Cauter E., Role of Sleep and Sleep Loss in Hormonal Release and Metabolism, Endocr. Dev. 17:11-21, 2010

217 Adámková V. et al., Association between duration of the sleep and body weight, Physiol. Res. 58 Suppl 1:S27-31, 2009

218 Patel S.R., Reduced sleep as an obesity risk factor, Obes, Rev. 10 Suppl 2:61-8, 2009

219 Thomas A. et al., Employees' sleep duration and body mass index: potential confounders, Prev. Med. 48(5):467-70, 2009

220 Padez C., Long sleep duration and childhood overweight/obesity and body fat, Am. J. Hum. Biol. 21(3):371-6, 2009

221 Park S.E. et al., The association between sleep duration and general and abdominal obesity in Koreans: data from the Korean National Health and Nutrition Examination Survey, 2001 and 2005, Obesity 17(4):767-71, 2009

222 Siervo M., Wells J.C., Cizza G., The contribution of psychosocial stress to the obesity epidemic: an evolutionary approach, Horm. Metab. Res. 41(4):261-70, 2009

223 Van Cauter E. et al., Metabolic consequences of sleep and sleep loss, Sleep Med. 9 Suppl 1:S23-8, 2008

224 Nedeltcheva A.V., Sleep curtailment is accompanied by increased intake of calories from snacks, Am. J. Clin. Nutr. 89(1):126-33, 2009

225 Touchette E. et al., Associations between sleep duration patterns and overweight/obesity at age 6, Sleep, 1;31(11):1507-14, 2008

226 Schmid S.M. et al., A single night of sleep deprivation increases ghrelin levels and feelings of hunger in normal-weight healthy men, J. Sleep Res. 17(3):331-4, 2008

227 Cappuccio F.P., Meta-analysis of short sleep duration and obesity in children and adults, Sleep 1;31(5):619-26, 2008

228 Wells J.C. et al., Sleep patterns and television viewing in relation to obesity and blood pressure: evidence from an adolescent Brazilian birth cohort, Int. J. Obes. 32(7):1042-9, 2008

229 Yu Y. et al., Short sleep duration and adiposity in Chinese adolescents, Sleep, 1;30(12):1688-97, 2007

230 Patel S.R., Hu F.B., Short sleep duration and weight gain: a systematic review, Obesity 16(3):643-53, 2008

231 Nixon G.M. et al., Short sleep duration in middle childhood: risk factors and consequences, Sleep 1;31(1):71-8, 2008

232 Buscemi D. et al., Short sleep times predict obesity in internal medicine clinic patients, J. Clin. Sleep Med. 15;3(7):681-8, 2007

233 Bosy-Westphal A. et al., Influence of partial sleep deprivation on energy balance and insulin sensitivity in healthy women, Obes. Facts. 1(5):266-273, 2008

234 Gunderson E.P. et al., Association of fewer hours of sleep at 6 months postpartum with substantial weight retention at 1 year postpartum, Am. J. Epidemiol. 15;167(2):178-87, 2008

235 Singh M. et al., The association between obesity and short sleep duration: a population-based study, J. Clin. Sleep Med. 15;1(4):357-63, 2005

236 Schmid S.M. et al., Sleep loss alters basal metabolic hormone secretion and modulates the dynamic counterregulatory response to hypoglycemia, J. Clin. Endocrinol. Metab. 92(8):3044-51, 2007

237 Knutson K.L. et al., The metabolic consequences of sleep deprivation, Sleep Med. Rev. 11(3):163-78, 2007

238 Gangwisch J.E., Epidemiological evidence for the links between sleep, circadian rhythms and metabolism, Obes. Rev. 10 Suppl 2:37-45, 2009

239 Copinschi G., Metabolic and endocrine effects of sleep deprivation, Essent. Psychopharmacol. 6(6):341-7, 2005

240 Seicean A. et al, Association between short sleeping hours and overweight in adolescents: results from a US Suburban High School survey, Sleep Breath 11(4):285-93, 2007

241 Toyoshima H. et al., Effect of the interaction between mental stress and eating pattern on body mass index gain in healthy Japanese male workers, J. Epidemiol. 19(2):88-93, 2009

242 Nishitani N., Sakakibara H., Akiyama I., Eating behavior related to obesity and job stress in male Japanese workers, Nutrition 25(1):45-50, 2009

243 Otsuka R. et al., Eating fast leads to obesity: findings based on self-administered questionnaires among middle-aged Japanese men and women, J. Epidemiol. 16(3):117-24, 2006

244 Sasaki S. et al., Self-reported rate of eating correlates with body mass index in 18-y-old Japanese women, Int. J. Obes. Relat. Metab. Disord. 27(11):1405-10, 2003

245 Otsuka R. et al., Eating fast leads to obesity: findings based on self-administered questionnaires among middle-aged Japanese men and women, J. Epidemiol. 16(3):117-24, 2006

246 Otsuka R. et al., Eating fast leads to insulin resistance: findings in middle-aged Japanese men and women, Prev. Med. 46(2):154-9, 2008

247 Cree M.G. et al., Twenty-eight-day bed rest with hypercortisolemia induces peripheral insulin resistance and increases intramuscular triglycerides, Metabolism 59(5):703-10, 2010

248 Vicennati V. et al., Stress-related development of obesity and cortisol in women, Obesity 17(9):1678-83, 2009

249 Roberts C. et al., The effects of stress on body weight: biological and psychological predictors of change in BMI, Obesity 15(12):3045-55, 2007

250 Bose M., Oliván B., Laferrère B., Stress and obesity: the role of the hypothalamic-pituitary-adrenal axis in metabolic disease, Curr. Opin. Endocrinol. Diabetes Obes. 16(5):340-6, 2009

251 Collison K.S. et al., Sugar-sweetened carbonated beverage consumption correlates with BMI, waist circumference, and poor dietary choices in school children, BMC Public Health 9;10:234, 2010

252 Babey S.H. et al., Bubbling over: soda consumption and its link to obesity in California, Policy Brief UCLA Cent Health Policy Res. (PB2009-5):1-8, 2009

253 Nissinen K. Et al., Sweets and sugar-sweetened soft drink intake in childhood in relation to adult BMI and overweight, The cardiovascular risk in young Finns study, Public Health Nutr. 12(11):2018-26, 2009

254 Mathern J.R. et al., Effect of fenugreek fiber on satiety, blood glucose and insulin response and energy intake in obese subjects, Phytother Res. 23(11):1543-8, 2009

255 Brown C.M., Dulloo A.G., Montani J.P., Sugary drinks in the pathogenesis of obesity and cardiovascular diseases, Int. J. Obes. 32 Suppl. 6:S28-34, 2008

256 Al-Waili N.S., Effects of daily consumption of honey solution on hematological indices and blood levels of minerals and enzymes in normal individuals, J. Med. Food 6(2):135-40, 2003

257 Chen L. et al., Reduction in consumption of sugar-sweetened beverages is associated with weight loss: the PREMIER trial, Am. J. Clin. Nutr. 89(5):1299-306, 2009

258 van Can J.G. et al., Reduced glycaemic and insulinaemic responses following isomaltulose ingestion: implications for postprandial substrate use, Br. J. Nutr. 102(10):1408-13, 2009

259 Bahrami M. et al., Effects of natural honey consumption in diabetic patients: an 8-week randomized clinical trial, Int. J. Food Sci. Nutr. 60(7):618-26, 2009

260 Yaghoobi N. et al., Natural honey and cardiovascular risk factors; effects on blood glucose, cholesterol, triacylglycerole, CRP, and body weight compared with sucrose, ScientificWorldJournal 20;8:463-9, 2008

261 Luoto R. et al., The impact of perinatal probiotic intervention on the development of overweight and obesity: follow-up study from birth to 10 years, Int. J. Obes. 16, 2010

262 Kadooka Y. et al., Regulation of abdominal adiposity by probiotics (Lactobacillus gasseri SBT2055) in adults with obese tendencies in a randomized controlled trial, Eur. J. Clin. Nutr. 10, 2010

263 Thuny F. et al., Vancomycin treatment of infective endocarditis is linked with recently acquired obesity, PLoS One 10;5(2):e9074, 2010

264 Luoto R. et al., Impact of maternal probiotic-supplemented dietary counselling on pregnancy outcome and prenatal and postnatal growth: a double-blind, placebo-controlled study, Br. J. Nutr. 4:1-8, 2010

265 Cani P.D., Delzenne N.M., The role of the gut microbiota in energy metabolism and metabolic disease, Curr. Pharm. Des. 15(13):1546-58, 2009

266 Hamad E.M. et al., Milk fermented by Lactobacillus gasseri SBT2055 influences adipocyte size via inhibition of dietary fat absorption in zucker rats, Br. J. Nutr. 101(5):716-24, 2009

267 Isolauri E. et al., Obesity – extending the hygiene hypothesis, Nestle Nutr. Workshop Ser. Pediatr. Program 64:75-85; discussion 85-9, 251-7, 2009

268 Lee K. et al., Antiobesity effect of trans-10, cis-12-conjugated linoleic acid-producing Lactobacillus plantarum PL62 on diet-induced obese mice, J. Appl. Microbiol. 103(4):1140-6, 2007

269 Kalliomäki M. et al., Early differences in fecal microbiota composition in children may predict overweight, Am. J. Clin. Nutr. 87(3):534-8, 2008

270 Lee H.Y. et al., Human originated bacteria, Lactobacillus rhamnosus PL60, produce conjugated linoleic acid and show anti-obesity effects in diet-induced obese mice, Biochim. Biophys. Acta. 1761(7):736-44, 2006

271 Tennyson C.A., Friedman G., Microecology, obesity, and probiotics, Curr. Opin. Endocrinol. Diabetes Obes. 15(5):422-7, 2008

272 DiBaise J.K., Gut microbiota and its possible relationship with obesity, Mayo. Clin. Proc. 83(4):460-9, 2008

273 Larsen N. et al., Gut microbiota in human adults with type 2 diabetes differs from non-diabetic adults, PLoS One 5;5(2):e9085, 2010

274 Schwiertz A. et al., Microbiota and SCFA in lean and overweight healthy subjects, Obesity 18(1):190-5, 2010

275 Borak J., Neonatal hypothyroidism due to maternal vegan diet, J. Pediatr. Endocrinol. Metab. 18(6):621, 2010

276 Pistelli F., Aquilini F., Carrozzi L., Weight gain after smoking cessation, Monaldi Arch. Chest Dis. 71(2):81-7, 2009

277 Deshpande A.D., et al., Epidemiology of diabetes and diabetes-related complications, Phys. Ther. 88(11):1254-64, 2008

278 Chiolero A. et al., Consequences of smoking for body weight, body fat distribution, and insulin resistance, Am. J. Clin. Nutr. 87(4):801-9, 2008

279 Stanworth R.D., Jones T.H., Testosterone for the aging male; current evidence and recommended practice, Clin. Interv. Aging 3(1): 25–44, 2008

280 Tishova Y., Kalinchenko S.Y., Breaking the vicious circle of obesity: the metabolic syndrome and low testosterone by administration of testosterone to a young man with morbid obesity, Arq. Bras. Endocrinol. Metabol. 53(8):1047-51, 2009

281 Andersen M.L., Tufik S., The effects of testosterone on sleep and sleep-disordered breathing in men: its bidirectional interaction with erectile function, Sleep Med. Rev. 12 (5): 365–79, 2008

282 Marin D.P., Figueira A.J. Junior, Pinto L.G., One session of resistance training may increase serum testosterone and triiodotironine in young men, Medicine & Science in Sports & Exercise 38 (5): S285, 2006

283 Armanini D. et al., Licorice reduces serum testosterone in healthy women, Steroids 69(11-12):763-6, 2004

284 Armanini D. et al., Licorice consumption and serum testosterone in healthy man, Exp. Clin. Endocrinol. Diabetes 111(6):341-3, 2003

285 Hermsdorff H.H., A legume-based hypocaloric diet reduces proinflammatory status and improves metabolic features in overweight/obese subjects, Eur. J. Nutr. 25, 2010

286 Gnacińska M. et al., Adipose tissue activity in relation to overweight or obesity, Endokrynol. Pol. 61(2):160-8, 2010

287 Kiecolt-Glaser J.K., Stress, food, and inflammation: psychoneuroimmunology and nutrition at the cutting edge, Psychosom. Med. 72(4):365-9. Epub 2010 Apr 21, 2010

288 Camargo A. et al., Gene expression changes in mononuclear cells in patients with metabolic syndrome after acute intake of phenol-rich virgin olive oil, BMC Genomics. 20;11:253, 2010

289 Wall R. et al., Fatty acids from fish: the anti-inflammatory potential of long-chain omega-3 fatty acids, Nutr. Rev. 68(5):280-9, 2010

290 Rayssiguier Y. et al., Magnesium deficiency and metabolic syndrome: stress and inflammation may reflect calcium activation, Magnes. Res. 31, 2010

291 Basu A., Rhone M., Lyons T.J., Berries: emerging impact on cardiovascular health, Nutr. Rev. 68(3):168-77, 2010

292 Heber D., An integrative view of obesity, Am. J. Clin. Nutr. 91(1):280S-283S, 2010

293 Adapala N., Chan M.M., Long-term use of an antiinflammatory, curcumin, suppressed type 1 immunity and exacerbated visceral leishmaniasis in a chronic experimental model, Lab. Invest. 88(12):1329-39, 2008

294 Astrup A. et al., Can bioactive foods affect obesity? Ann. NY Acad. Sci. 1190; 25-41, 2010

295 Zemel M.B. et al., Calcium and diary acceleration of weight and fat loss during energy restriction in obese adults, Obes. Res. 12:582-590, 2004

296 Zemel M.B. et al., Diary augmentation of total and central fat loss in obese subjects, Int. J. Obes. 29:391-397, 2005

297 Ohman M. et al., Biochemical effects of consumption of eggs containing omega-3 polyunsaturated fatty acids, Ups. J. Med. Sci. 113(3):315-23, 2008

298 Boston B.A., The role of melanocortins in adipocyte function, Ann. N Y Acad. Sci. 20;885:75-84, 1999

299 Cettour-Rose P., Rohner-Jeanrenaud F., The leptin-like effects of 3-d peripheral administration of a melanocortin agonist are more marked in genetically obese Zucker (fa/fa) than in lean rats, Endocrinology 143(6):2277-83, 2002

300 Hwa J.J. et al., Central melanocortin system modulates energy intake and expenditure of obese and lean Zucker rats, Am. J. Physiol. Regul. Integr. Comp. Physiol. 281(2):R444-51, 2001

301 Chen A.S. et al., Role of the melanocortin-4 receptor in metabolic rate and food intake in mice, Transgenic Res. 9(2):145-54, 2000

302 Pierroz D.D. et al., Effects of acute and chronic administration of the melanocortin agonist MTII in mice with diet-induced obesity, Diabetes 51(5):1337-45, 2002

303 Krotkiewski M., Thyroid hormones in the pathogenesis and treatment of obesity, Eur. J. Pharmacol. 12;440(2-3):85-98, 2002

304 Broberger C., Hökfelt T., Peptider öppnar för nya behandlingar av övervikt och aptitlöshet, Läkartidningen 49, Vol 99, s. 4982-4989, 2002

305 Katcher H.I. et al. The effects of a whole grain enriched hypocaloric diet on cardiovascular disease risk factors in men and women with metabolic syndrome, Am. J. Clin. Nutr. 87: 79-90, 2008

306 Wisker E. et al., Digestibilities of energy, protein, fat and nonstarch polysaccharides in a low fiber diet and diets containing coarse or fine whole meal rye are comparable in rats and humans, J. Nutr. 126: 481-488, 1996

307 Chen H.L. et al., Mechanisms by which wheat bran and oat bran increase stool weight in humans, Am. J. Clin. Nutr. 68: 711-719, 1998

308 Rigaud D. et al., Effects of a moderate dietary fibre supplement on hunger rating, energy input and feacal energy output in young, healthy volunteers, A randomized, double-blind, cross-over trial, Int. J. Obes. 11 (Suppl 1): 73-78, 1987

309 Walters R.L. et al., Effects of two types of fibre on faecal steroid and lipid excretion, Br. Med. J. 2: 536-538, 1975

310 Ganji V., Kies C.V., Psyllium husk fibre supplementation to soybean and coconut oil diets of humans: effect on fat digestibility and faecal fatty acid excretion, Eur. J. Clin. Nutr. 48: 595-597, 1994

311 Miles C.W., Kelsay J.L., Wong N.P., Effect of dietary fiber on the metabolizable energy of human diets, J. Nutr. 118: 1075-1081, 1988

312 Adam T.C., Westerterp-Plantenga M.S., Glucagon-like peptide-1 release and satiety after a nutrient challenge in normal-weight and obese subjects, Br. J. Nutr. 93: 845-851, 2005

313 Samra R.A., Anderson G.H., Insoluble cereal fiber reduces appetite and short-term food intake and glycemic response to food consumed 75 min later by healthy men, Am. J. Clin. Nutr. 86; 972-979, 2007

314 Berti C. et al., Effect on appetite control of minor cereal and pseudocereal products, Br. J. Nutr. 94: 850-858, 2005

315 Johnston K.L. et al., Resistant starch improves insulin sensitivity in metabolic syndrome, Diabet. Med. 27(4):391-7, 2010

316 Higgins J.A. et al., Resistant starch consumption promotes lipid oxidation, Nutr. Metab. 6;1(1):8, 2004

317 Nichols J., Ross S., Patterson P., Thermic effect of food at rest and following swim exercise in trained college men and wome, Ann. Nutr. Metab. 32(4):215-9, 1988

318 Lavin J.H., French S.J., Read N.W., The effect of sucrose- and aspartame-sweetened drinks on energy intake, hunger and food choice of female, moderately restrained eaters, Int. J. Obes. Relat. Metab. Disord. 21(1):37-42, 1997

319 Fischer-Posovszky P. et al., Resveratrol regulates human adipocyte number and function in a Sirt1-dependent manner1,2,3, Am. J. Clin. Nutr. 92: 5-15, 2010

320 Barr S.B., Wright J.C., Postprandial energy expenditure in whole-food and processed-food meals: implications for daily energy expenditure, Food & Nutrition Research Vol 54, 2010